Praise for *Bravey*

"Vulnerable. Honest. Powerful. *Bravey* is the kind of book I want to tell my friends about, recommend to strangers, and one day encourage my daughter to read. Pappas is an incredible storyteller whose willingness to delve into the scary parts of life makes *Bravey* an important read."

—Allyson Felix, Olympic gold medalist

"Alexi Pappas has turned unimaginable loss and pain into an engine for empathy, uniqueness, and excellence. I've always believed that your greatest tragedy can become your greatest strength, and Alexi Pappas is living proof. Be brave, read *Bravey,* be a Bravey."

—Jay Duplass, filmmaker and author of *Like Brothers*

"Wise and beautiful . . . After surviving a gritty, jaw-clenching 2020, *Bravey* feels like a giant exhale."

—*Women's Running*

"A thoughtful, beautiful read; breathtakingly honest and poignantly insightful."

—*Refinery29*

"*Bravey* will make you laugh, while also inspiring readers to reject the limitations society seeks to impose on us."

—*PopSugar* ("Best Books of January 2021")

"Vulnerable, real, motivating."

—*A Cup of Jo*

"[*Bravey* is] a fitting title for her memoir. I think of Alexi Pappas as someone fiercely focused on hugely ambitious external goals. But in this book, she turns that focus inward to examine her childhood, her family, and her own mind."

—Ari Shapiro, NPR's *All Things Considered*

"Inspiring . . . delightful . . . a wise blueprint for all the rest of us to become [a] bravey too."

—*People* ("The Best New Books")

"[Pappas] writes with a poet's economy of word and a filmmaker's grasp of narrative."

—*Runner's World*

"Pappas approaches mental health issues with a fresh and thoughtful mindset, evidence that she's done the hard work of processing her trauma and has come out the other side with more self-love and self-knowledge than ever before. Readers—whether they're athletes or not—are sure to find her mental health takeaways helpful."

—*Shondaland*

"In her excellent new memoir *Bravey,* Alexi dives deeper. An exuberant and unflinching primer on the struggle of self-actualization, it's the beautiful story of surviving trauma and navigating disparate dreams—filmmaking and athletics—in competition for her attention. Why she refused to pick just one lane. And how, setbacks and deep lows aside, Alexi ultimately succeeds at both."

—Rich Roll, *The Rich Roll Podcast*

"[A] cross-domain talent . . . Pappas incisively recounts emotional highs and lows."

—*Psychology Today*

"Through perseverance and diligence, Alexi is a multi-talented force to be reckoned with, as she has taken her experiences from the Olympic podium and has strategically presented her knowledgeable ideals into her newest book, *Bravey*."

—*Noemi*

"In *Bravey,* Pappas says all she's ever wanted in her life is to matter. And matter she does, with this dazzling memoir-in-essays, as well as the lived experiences behind them all. Pappas is an intuitively skilled writer, a born storyteller. . . . *Bravey* is a much-needed dose of motivation, inspiration, and encouragement to stick to it and continue following your own dreams, even—and perhaps especially—when you are scared."

—*The Nerd Daily*

"*Bravey* confronts both loss and triumph, comedy and sadness. It is peppered with [Pappas's] poetry and prose, making it uniquely her own. Not only does *Bravey* offer a window into the mind of an Olympian, but the reader watches Pappas grow up in real time."

—*The Daily Californian*

"In this strong debut, Olympian Pappas shares her inspiring life story of overcoming tragedy as a child to enjoy a flourishing, multifaceted career as an athlete, filmmaker, and actor. . . . Pappas's extraordinary tale is skillfully told and profoundly inspiring."

—*Publishers Weekly*

"A celebrity running memoir on the outside; on the inside, an instruction manual for thriving based on a lifetime of hardearned wisdom. Add writing to Pappas's domains of success. . . . From the first page, Pappas is vulnerable, honest, and courageous—not to mention funny. Whether writing about social awkwardness, professional disappointments, or her mother's suicide, she maintains a buoyant spirit that becomes wonderfully contagious. . . . Inspiring, yes, but more to the point: genuinely empowering. An utterly winning collection of personal essays."

—*Kirkus Reviews* (starred review)

"This is not only an inspiring look inside the mind of a gifted athlete—it's an arresting debut by a gifted writer. Alexi Pappas reveals how we can find the courage to face our fears, the grit to achieve our goals, and the resilience to bounce forward after failure and heartbreak. I couldn't put it down."

—Adam Grant, #1 *New York Times* bestselling author of *Originals*

"*Bravey* is at once a memoir of an inspiring young life-in-progress and a practical how-to manual of willpower and overcoming. It's about dealing with the life you're born into and have little control over, and the larger quest for the greatest expression of oneself. *Bravey* is also a unique articulation of the necessary dual tracks of visualizing a reality and imagining your life into existence, along with all the hard work and the commitment that is required. Wish I could have read it as a younger person!"

—Richard Linklater, Academy Award–nominated director

"Like a sort of human Möbius strip, Alexi Pappas has the ability to turn the pain and loss she's experienced in her life into a tool for repairing that pain and loss. And then to repair yours. Or rather, to help you repair yours—she has strong feelings that we all need to learn things for ourselves. This is no glib, triumphal memoir of overcoming adversity. Pappas is a genuine and vulnerable narrator, and as she fledges from nest after nest, she makes plenty of falls. Like any story about real human growth, hers is not linear or neat. But through it all she stays open to what comes next—as good a description of what it means to be brave as I've ever heard."

—Alison Bechdel,
New York Times bestselling author of *Fun Home*

"*Bravey* heralds the debut of a skilled memoirist. In heartfelt, vibrant prose, Alexi Pappas gives us her captivating life story. A beautiful read that is sure to resonate deeply."

—Ruth Reichl,
New York Times bestselling author of *Save Me the Plums*

"*Bravey* made me laugh out loud, brought me to tears, and gave me so many mantras I now live by. Alexi Pappas not only has a powerful way with words, but also uses the stories and lessons in this beautiful book as an intimate view into who she is. If you read this book, then you know Alexi Pappas, and knowing her is truly a gift."

— Mary Cain, World Junior Champion runner

"If you need a shot of courage, resilience, and motivation, look no further than *Bravey*. Alexi Pappas's fearlessness and inner power offer a guide for how we can all step into the lives we most desire. Honest and propulsive, *Bravey* shows how we can overcome past traumas to run whatever our race might be—and we know we will have Pappas rooting for us."

— Tara Schuster, author of *Buy Yourself the F*cking Lilies*

"With *Bravey,* Alexi Pappas tells a story of persevering through hardship, finding your footing as a leader, and harnessing the unrivaled power of teamwork. Her book, which is candid, funny, and real, offers practical guidance to those looking to forge through obstacles, build their teams, and become leaders in their own lives."

— Abby Wambach, #1 *New York Times* bestselling author of *Wolfpack*

"I think there is a reason why we encounter certain books in life. I was awed by Alexi Pappas's beautiful memoir *Bravey*. It resonated so deeply with me that at times it felt like Pappas was inside my own head. Her story shows us how to build mental strength and what it means for superheroes to make their own capes. *Bravey* offers essential guidance to anyone dreaming big dreams."

—Shalane Flanagan, Olympic silver medalist,
NYC Marathon winner, and *New York Times* bestselling
author of *Run Fast. Eat Slow.*

"Pappas's heartbreaking and hilarious book inspired even *me* to want to put on some sneakers and run."

—Mindy Kaling,
#1 *New York Times* bestselling author of *Why Not Me?*

BRAVEY

BRAVEY

Chasing Dreams, Befriending Pain,
and Other Big Ideas

ALEXI PAPPAS
FOREWORD BY MAYA RUDOLPH

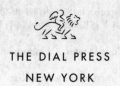

THE DIAL PRESS

NEW YORK

2022 Dial Press Trade Paperback Edition

Published in the United States by The Dial Press, an imprint of Random House,
a division of Penguin Random House LLC, New York.

THE DIAL PRESS is a registered trademark and the colophon is a trademark of
Penguin Random House LLC.
RANDOM HOUSE BOOK CLUB and colophon are trademarks of
Penguin Random House LLC.

Originally published in hardcover in the United States by The Dial Press, an
imprint of Random House, a division of Penguin Random House LLC, in 2021.

"My Pal, Pain" was originally published in different form in
Lenny Letter, August 17, 2016.

Trade paperback ISBN 978-1-9848-0114-2
Ebook ISBN 978-1-9848-0113-5

Printed in the United States of America on acid-free paper

randomhousebooks.com
randomhousebookclub.com

2 4 6 8 9 7 5 3 1

Book design by Diane Hobbing

This book is for Dad. I think we did it.

CONTENTS

FOREWORD

By Maya Rudolph

I have spent the majority of my life making people laugh. Well, at least trying to. I remember when I was around seven years old, I was playing with a friend when she got hurt and started to cry. I felt so uncomfortable in that moment of seeing her in pain that I immediately thought of the quickest route to avoidance: laughter. I proceeded to do a goofy voice and threw in a pratfall for good measure—and lo and behold, it worked. She forgot her pain, and I didn't have to deal with what pain feels like. Avoiding feelings like pain and sadness came naturally to me.

If I had to guess, I would probably attribute this to my own childhood trauma, having lost my mother to breast cancer right before my seventh birthday. Just a hunch. It's safe to say most comedians share this wildly attractive trait. You know that old chestnut about how comedians all have the same black hole in their hearts due to sadness? It's probably true.

Comedy is a wonderful avoidance tool that I would highly recommend if you're not up for feeling your feelings. It's a mask you can wear, a suit of armor you can don to protect the very mushy parts of your insides too fragile to embrace. But I think the most interesting part about comedy is that it is a manipulation. A sleight of hand to distract you from the dark, ugly stuff. This tool has served me well over the years, but there are just some things in life you can't throw a joke at. You have to face them head on.

During what felt like a particularly low point in my adult life, when I had to make a tough decision, a good friend asked me, "You know the definition of *brave,* right?" And she went on to say, "It's facing your fears," or maybe she said, "Being strong even though you're scared," or . . . wait a minute, I think I wrote down what she said so that I wouldn't forget it . . . aaaand I can't find it. So I looked up the definition of *brave* in the dictionary and it reads as follows:

Brave—ready to face and endure danger or pain; showing courage.

Courage, huh? Hmm, interesting. Then I figured I would look up the true meaning of *courage,* which is, after all, at the root of bravery:

Courage—the ability to do something that frightens one; strength in the face of pain or grief.

And if we wanted to get really deep, the root of the word *courage* comes from the Latin root word, *cor,* which then became the French word *coeur,* meaning "heart."

Courage makes me think of Bert Lahr's Cowardly Lion in *The Wizard of Oz.* Over years of watching this movie many times, I realized he was my least favorite of the new friends Dorothy met along the yellow brick road. And honestly, I think it was because he was such a wuss. Scarecrow's lack of intellect was charming next to some incredible dance moves, and who couldn't fall for a guy made out of tin who just wanted to feel love with a real heart? But when I got to the Lion I thought, *God, this guy's a real crybaby.* But here's the thing: He was really funny.

I would only find out years later, from experience, that the funny guy was actually the guy you wanted to be in the movie. Sure, the Scarecrow danced pretty and the Tin Man was a charmer but the Lion was the one who got to be big and vulnerable, and those are the juiciest roles to play because they are grounded in reality, which can ultimately be so deeply painful. Not only did the Lion really have the courage he was seeking all along, his courage was deeply rooted in heart. He had no idea his courage was always there, he just didn't see it. Because he told himself it wasn't there.

So why do we do this to ourselves? Why don't we see ourselves the way others do? It is so much easier to name greatness outside of ourselves. This is true of my first impressions of Alexi Pappas. Encountering an Olympian is an otherworldly experience in and of itself. It feels like the closest thing to standing next to a superhero. There is, of course, the obvious physical difference between us—her body can do things we mere mortals are not capable of—but it is also my belief that her greatness doesn't just manifest in her physical form, you also witness it at the mental level.

Over the years working at *Saturday Night Live,* people often asked me who my favorite hosts were and without hesitation

I've always said the professional athletes. (Derek Jeter to name one.) And I think it is because of the incredibly calm, almost blissfully sedated ease that they carry themselves with. It's a sort of "I can do anything" demeanor. Hosting a live television show isn't scary to Derek Jeter because hitting a home run to left field in front of a crowd of 50,000 people is just a day at work for him.

I assume this superhuman level of nirvana-like steadiness can be attributed to the body's release of dopamine and endorphins as a result of regular exercise that makes athletes just feel happy—or, in Jeter's case, cool and super-smooth. I wouldn't know, considering during my time at *SNL* I was happily doing just the opposite: putting in fourteen-hour days and pulling all-nighters writing at 30 Rock, then doing a weekly live television show that didn't start until 11:30 P.M., didn't end until 1:00 A.M., and then there was the after-party that started at 1:30, which meant Sundays were shot, and sometimes I would only get out of bed as the sun was going down just to order Chinese food and then get back into bed. Not exactly the profile of a professional athlete.

So this brings me back to Alexi. My initial assumption was that this superior being in human form somehow possessed all of life's answers because of her (what I believed to be) superhuman prowess. But this was just something I created as a justification for my own self-consciousness. This isn't to say that Alexi isn't remarkable; in fact, she is. But the pedestal that I created for her is really just a smokescreen for the truth: That underneath it all, all human beings are vulnerable at our core. And that it is in the power of the individual to create one's own destiny.

Children of trauma know this all too well. We go through life

thinking everyone else has it better than us until we grow up
and realize we're all in our own tiny boats of self-doubt and
second-guessing. (This is probably why puberty was invented.
To humiliate us all and bring us all down to the same level so
that we'd just grow the fuck up. The great equalizer!) My dad
loved to share the adage that if you got everyone in the world
together to put all their problems into one giant pot, everyone
would just end up taking their own problems back. But what
about the smaller percentage of us who lost parents and felt like
we weren't "normal"? The weirdos who desperately just wanted
to have straight hair and tiny noses so we could skate through
life unnoticed because we were so tired of "And how old were
you when your mother died? Oh, that must have been so hard
for you." Or was that just me?

But then as we grow up something interesting happens.
Somehow we manage to find each other. To connect and actually become the new normal: broken but not defeated, and glued
back together again and again and again. I think this is such a
clear testament to the human spirit. We have an endless capacity
to grow and surprise ourselves, and it is amazing what we can
accomplish, from little things we never thought we could do on
upward.

For me, that little thing was roasting a chicken. It seemed like
such an intimidating recipe, filled to the brim with risk of sal-
monella poisoning. Roasting a chicken was something that
mothers do, real moms, ones who make their first attempt under
the careful supervision of their own moms, adult hands cupping
the outside of their own. A lesson I never received, thereby making me dangerously unqualified to roast a chicken for my own
family. But one day I set my fear of failure aside and finally just

tried it. And now I'm a master. Not Alice Waters level or anything but the kind that feels triumphant and exudes confidence.
There is such a calm relief in knowing you can count on yourself. Sure, sometimes you'd rather curl up in a ball and let someone else take care of you while you throw your own pity party,
but that chicken's not going to roast itself. And guess what? You
tried and you didn't die. And life goes on. And if we're lucky, on
and on.

Alexi, what you have shared here is no less than brave. It is
incredibly human and vulnerable and shows an uncompromis-
ing spirit. And what makes it so deeply personal is what makes
it so relatable. I am grateful to have found you and to be able
to hold a mirror up for you the way your courage has done for
me. Thank you for sharing your beautiful aches and pains and
triumphs with all of us. I still believe that you are superhuman,
but that is truly because of who you are. Your ability to examine
your life is a generous gift. You are a true Bravey. And since
reading this book, I can now confidently say that I am a Bravey,
too.

Your friend,
Maya

BRAVEY

Introduction

BE A BRAVEY

My earliest memory of running was in the first grade when a boy in my class made fun of my best friend, and I not only chased him down but caught him and stabbed him with a pencil to make sure he knew I wasn't fucking around. In middle school I channeled my athletic ability in a more productive way: the track team. Organized chasing. We had weekly meets at the local high-school dirt track, which was very exciting to us twelve-year-olds. The meets were coed and I won them all. I liked the feeling of winning. It made me feel like I mattered. All I've ever wanted in my life is to matter.

* * *

I was born in Berkeley, and I grew up in a safe slice of suburbia outside of San Francisco with my remarkable father and loving older brother. But despite the privilege and security of my up-bringing, my bright future was not guaranteed. My first five years of life coincided with my mom's last. Shortly after I came into the world my mom became so mentally ill that she had to be hospitalized. For all I know, I was the last straw that sent her over the edge. I am always saddened by the sense that I came at just the wrong time.

She was diagnosed as bipolar with manic depression, and after developing an addiction to pain pills originally prescribed to treat a back injury due to pregnancy complications, she became suicidal—unsuccessfully at first and then, eventually, successfully. But my mom succeeded in other things long before she succeeded at suicide. She was an accomplished athlete and one of the first female software consultants at her company. What I now understand is that a successful person can be successful in anything, the good and the bad. This is both empowering and heartbreaking.

Living with my mom for my first five years of childhood forced me to learn how to survive in a different way. I had an awareness of just how extreme life can be. Like all kids, the thing I wanted most in the world was attention. But when you're a toddler and the person throwing temper tantrums in your house is your mom instead of you, attention is hard to come by. It was easy to feel like I didn't matter.

When I saw how my dad and the parade of doctors were always crowding around my mom and paying attention to her, my four-year-old brain could only think: Why don't people pay attention to *me* like that? It wasn't that my dad didn't want to give me all the attention in the world, it was just that he couldn't. All of my early memories, even the happy ones, are tinted with this feeling that I'm the least interesting thing in the room.

Mattering taunted me because it felt like it was not for me. I remember feeling desperate to do whatever it took to get the attention I craved. And so I decided that I would need to become the most interesting thing in the room. I decided that even though I didn't matter enough for my mom to choose to stay with me, I would matter to everyone else. I would become great. I translated my internal desires into external effort. I would learn, in time, how painful and unsustainable it is to be fueled by trauma like this. But I am where I am because of it.

* * *

In those early middle school years, whether I won a race or not was purely a question of how hard I could push myself. It was a contest of me versus my own pain tolerance. This is why I love to run. Because it is a way for me to push on and explore the outermost limits of myself, mentally and physically, in a way that is fundamentally good. That basic principle has held true throughout my running career, from my time as a young natural to when I was the worst on my college team all the way up to competing in the Olympics. The same dynamic applies to my creative pursuits: How much pain, how much uncertainty, how much discomfort am I brave enough to endure before I give up? Being brave is the best way to survive, and I've always been about survival.

As I grew into a decorated college athlete and then into an Olympian (with some major ups and downs along the way), I began to attract a modest but loyal following of younger athletes on social media. However small my audience was at first, I was keenly aware that being a role model is a privilege and a responsibility. When I was growing up, I sought out female role models shamelessly, watched them wide-eyed, and leaned on them hard. The best tools are the ones you have with you, not the ones you don't, and as a motherless daughter I have always been very forthcoming about my desire for mentorship. I idolized Mia Hamm and I mailed fan letters to the Spice Girls; the girls on the Cal Berkeley women's soccer team were like gods to me. I looked up to my friends' mothers, my college professors, and then, as I began my running career and making movies, I looked up to Olympians and artists.

I knew there would be kids, much like the little girl I had once been, who would pore over every word I posted and try their best to imitate it. I didn't want them trying to replicate my hundred-plus-miles-a-week training regimen; I wanted to give them something they could healthily adopt as their own. So instead of posting workout splits, I posted poems.

The poems were whimsical, silly thoughts, sometimes from the perspective of a runner but just as often from the perspective of two shoes in love or a trail that misses the runner after she's gone. One night, before a particularly daunting workout, I typed out this poem:

> *run like a bravey*
> *sleep like a baby*
> *dream like a crazy*
> *replace can't with maybe*

It was the first time I used the word *bravey*, and it stuck. It became the label for a mini-movement, a self-identifier for those who are willing to chase their dreams even though it can be intimidating and scary. It celebrates the choice to pursue a goal and even relishes the pain that comes with effort. There is nobility to it; it's something to be celebrated.

Growing up, I chased specific labels: strong, fierce, fast, funny, pretty. But all of those labels were *outward facing*—they described an energy you project into the world. Being a Bravey is different. It's *inward facing*, a choice you make about your relationship with yourself. We all have dreams that we're chasing, however big or small, and we can all decide to be brave enough to give ourselves a chance. I think that's why the term resonated with so many people: Anyone can be a Bravey, and the permutations of what that means are infinite. It's a switch you flip in your mind.

* * *

In writing a book about chasing dreams, I am, in fact, chasing one of my dreams: to write something that I know will *matter*, to you and to me. Chasing a dream is a never-ending negotiation, as in, you have to keep navigating, pivoting, adapting, and persisting. It's a process that unfolds continually and never in a straight line.

So much of my own growth was thanks to the mentors who, whether knowingly or unknowingly, let me learn from them. Now it is my turn. To really matter to those who might look up to me, I need to share my full story. I need to hold a magnifying glass up to the moments in my life when I was growing into myself.

This book is about glamorous things like going to the Olympics and making movies, and it's also about difficult things like suicide and depression and puberty. For every fun moment of victory in this book, there are uncomfortable and humiliating moments, too. I am the sum of all of them. I want to show you the whole picture, the bad pain and the good pain. This book is gore and glory. This book is about making a life, not just living a life. We will grow up together here.

A life can't be replicated and it doesn't need to be. But by sharing my story so far, I can show you what being a Bravey means to me. In turn, you can decide what being a Bravey means to you.

good thing i didn't accomplish all my goals yet

because then what would i do tomorrow?

FOUR MEMORIES OF MY MOTHER

I used to feed the ducks that lived in the lagoon behind our house. My dad went with me sometimes, but most often I went alone—the lagoon bordered our backyard and it was easy for me to slip away undetected. My favorite day to feed the ducks was Saturday, which was when moms and daughters were out in force. I'm sure other people were out there, too, but I have always cared most about moms and daughters.

Moms were aliens to me, foreign creatures I could only see outside of my home. I'd observe them from my vantage point atop a pile of wood chips as they walked down the bike path along the lagoon's edge. Obsessively watching those women was a compulsion stronger than being glued to Saturday-morning cartoons.

The moms would always walk with a bag of stale bread in one hand and their daughter's small hand in the other. I so badly wanted to experience that feeling of having my hand held by a woman who was walking half a step ahead of me. Wherever she was going, we'd head there together.

The mom-daughter duos all blend together in my mind: the daughter watching as the mom separates pieces of stale bread for her to throw into the water, as if the child can't tear up bread on her own. If the ducks ever got too close for comfort, the mom would swoop in, a protector shielding her precious youngling from the squawking assailants. She'd shoo the scary ducks away and then crouch down and look at her little girl closely, their faces in a vacuum away from the rest of the world, and tell her that everything was okay. She'd wipe the tears off her daughter's cheeks and brush the wood chips off her daughter's ankles as if to make her whole again. It didn't even seem like it was a special occasion that the daughter was being comforted by her mother; it was as natural and innocuous as breathing. In those moments I wanted very badly to climb into the bubble they created, to feel the warm air inside. I felt resentful but still curious, unable to look away, like when you're little and you have to watch your brother open presents on his birthday.

I liked to watch how the moms talked to other moms, acting as translators if their kids wanted to add anything to the conversation, always so understanding of each other, nodding and smiling and laughing. I thought maybe my mom didn't realize she could have gone to the park to find people to talk to.

I liked how the moms would listen to their children's overly descriptive monologues as if they were sharing critical information before the mom would tactfully decide whether or not to insert her own wisdom. One of the most common exchanges was when a kid would tell their mom they were hungry, but when the mom would offer healthy snacks like apple slices or celery sticks, the kid would say NO to all of these options so the mom would counter with, "Well then, you must not be very hungry after all!" Then a negotiation would ensue, and the kid and the mom would come to an agreement on the ratio of apple slices to gummy worms the child was allowed to eat. I never negotiated with my dad for anything and I had no idea how these kids could negotiate with their mothers—what leverage could a child possibly have? I would have gladly eaten those apples with the cores already cut out!

Every little girl watches and looks up to the older women in her orbit. There's an innate desire to admire them and to want to be like them. I know this because my cousin and I used to spy on my aunt while she was getting ready to go out to dinner, imitating her with our fingers as she strapped on her bra. Little girls linger while their mom is on the phone with her friends, soaking in the gossip that they'll most definitely misinterpret and regurgitate to their friends. Little girls stand very close and watch their moms in the bathroom stall at the airport. They look closely at their moms while their moms clean them up. These are looks of deep need, as if their mothers always *make everything okay*.

I imagine all little girls as potatoes, wondrous nuggets of raw potential just waiting to be shaped by their mom-chefs. Whether your mom tenderly styles you into a Hasselback dish, tosses you in the microwave, or is totally absent, she is going to affect you. My mother took her own life before there was much time for her to shape me into anything. I was four years old, almost five. The greatest legacy she left me was her suicide. I try to imagine what it feels like to be washed, dried, peeled—to be turned over under warm water, then pushed gently into an oven and basted every now and again. But it is another thing entirely to never be touched at all; to be left alone in the cabinet to sprout eyes and fend for yourself.

* * *

Before she died, my mother was in and out of my life like a jack-in-the-box. By the time I was four years old I knew she was sick, I just didn't understand quite what that meant. At that age, sick meant a sneeze or maybe an ear infection. It had easy-to-spot symptoms and was cured by taking gooey sweet red medicine. But none of that applied to my mother's mental illness. Depression is an invisible disease. Back then people generally didn't understand that depression is an illness like any other. Depression is something that you *have,* not something that you *are*. The stigma around depression begins with the way we talk about it and the way we label it. But I didn't understand this as a kid. I was looking for sneezes but all I saw were screams.

My mother had to be kept in a special place, locked up, safe from herself. But even there she was not entirely safe. According to her medical reports, she once lit her room and herself on fire. The orderlies caught her and she did not die that day. What do you need to feel inside to light yourself on fire? Do you feel fire inside that you need to get out, or do you feel nothing inside and so maybe lighting your hospital bed on fire and lying down in it is the only thing that can make you feel something? I was brought to visit her the way you'd visit someone in jail, in a highly controlled and scheduled way, but I don't remember anything other than the sterile white walls and fluorescent lights.

My mother was deeply mysterious to me. In my mind's eye she was very tall, which is funny because I later learned she was well under five feet. I'm actually much taller now than she was, but even so, in all of my imagined scenarios where I meet her again she is still somehow taller than me. She used to wear swooshy nylon sweat suits with matching pants and a jacket. I cannot remember her ever wearing anything but these matching sweat suits. When I wear matching sweat suits now, it is a secret nod to her.

Sometimes my mother was allowed to come home. This was a highly anticipated event in my family. It meant she had demonstrated enough outward-facing progress to be released from the asylum. Even as a toddler I could tell it was a very big deal, like when a dad buys fresh lobster for the entire family, one for everyone. It's a special occasion! But when my mother came home it never felt like she belonged there. I remember knowing *in theory* how moms and daughters were supposed to embrace and feel at ease with each other, but I was never able to actually achieve this with my mother. I don't remember ever hugging her. I'm sure she sensed this awkwardness, too, which must have made it even harder for her to come home—especially when it meant coming home to my brother and me, two little potatoes who were growing and transforming wildly, always one step more evolved than the last time she saw us. I imagine that she must have felt increasingly alienated from us and maybe even started thinking that it would be better if she were gone.

Even though her goal with suicide might have been to disappear, there are things about her I will never be able to forget. I have four memories of my mother and three of them are bad. They sit in the back of my mind all the time, like a lady on a green velvet chaise longue who mostly blends into the background but will sometimes wink and wave at me to get my attention. I remember she is there at all the wrong times. I am learning, slowly, to simply wave back.

* * *

In my earliest memory of my mother, she's leaning against the doorframe of the office in our old house wearing a red edition of the nylon sweat suit and smoking a cigarette. I still think of her anytime I smell cigarette smoke. My dad never told her not to smoke inside the house, even though I could see it bothered him. I figured that she was allowed because she was special. She stood in the doorway staring into nowhere, totally motionless save for the cigarette. Her hair, which was short and curly, absorbed the smoke around her. She looked like a movie poster to me, grainy and glamorous and ethereal, not all the way there. In college, girls on drugs who smoked cigarettes in fraternity basements looked like my memory of my mother: tragic and theatrical, beautiful and standoffish. People have a certain demeanor when they're smoking cigarettes, like they're listening to a story they've heard before, as if they'd rather be out there, somewhere else. Their hands are occupied and so is their mouth; they are not able to hold your hand or kiss you.

My mother and I were home alone—my dad tried to be there to supervise as much as he could, but sometimes he had to leave. This was always a roll of the dice for him, since he never knew what she was going to do next, ever. Her behavior ranged from compulsively buying things, like several life-size wooden parrot statuettes that she hung throughout the house, to totaling our family's minivan (possibly on purpose). Thankfully, I was not in the car when she wrecked it, but they found the car seat dangling upside down because it had not been secured properly. She was like a natural disaster and my dad was on alert all the time, never sure when her next episode was coming and how severe it would be—all the while balancing a full-time job, taking care of my brother and me, and managing my mom's care while keeping her condition a secret. Her stays at home always ended abruptly with her needing to be committed to some hospital, whether it was the psych ward or a rehab clinic or I don't know where else.

My mother was mesmerizing to me. I watched her smoke her cigarette and then I walked up next to her, almost close enough to touch her, though I don't remember actually touching her, *ever*. She was like a mean house cat that occasionally and very randomly permits you to approach. When she was really still like this and in one of her very quiet moods, I could get close. I have always been so jealous of little girls who dangle from their moms' thighs like jungle gyms. It still makes me ache in a way that is hard to admit when I see a little girl latched onto her mom like a snail on a leaf. I know that I would have loved this privilege and exercised it often.

I inched closer to my mother, almost close enough to feel the swooshy nylon against my skin, and then all of a sudden she came to life. She looked down at me as though I were a problem she didn't quite know how to solve. It wasn't mean but it wasn't nice. It was almost curious. She paused, took a drag of her cigarette, and then did something I don't remember her ever having done before: She reached her arm out to me. The caramel-brown mouthpiece was inches from my lips, and just out of focus was the bright hot point with smoke tendrils curling up to the ceiling. I understood she was offering me a puff. She didn't make a big deal of holding the cigarette in front of my mouth. It felt casual, almost like an accident—except it wasn't. I immediately felt special. The rules did not apply to us. I was her daughter and she was sharing something with me that had touched her lips and soon would touch mine. I felt like I was included in an exclusive thing that I had only ever seen her doing alone.

She held the cigarette to my mouth and I did what I had seen her do. I watched her as I did it, like how a baby might look into her mother's eyes as she breast-feeds. I inhaled shyly. The smoke was curiously harsh, like nothing I'd ever tasted before. I was used to soft things like chocolate milk and macaroni and cheese. I sensed that what was happening was not normal, that we were breaking a rule, but still I did it. I wanted her to love me more than I wanted to be good. I wanted her to include me. Who behaves crazier, a mentally ill person or a four-year-old who desperately wants her mother's love? When the most important person in your life is floating away like a ghost, you seize any opportunity you can to feel a connection with her. So of course I smoked the cigarette, even though I knew that smoking was B-A-D bad.

This cigarette is the only gift I remember ever receiving from my mom. But when she was away at the hospital, I'd take things that were hers and "give" them to myself. I took her lipstick and tried it on, wanting to see if it would make me look more like the woman I imagined I might one day become. I had ideas from Disney movies about what I might look like when I grew up. These days I wear ball gowns and high heels and full makeup far less often than the Disney princesses I once idolized, but back then they were my only guideposts. I took my mother's mink coat and wore it around the house with nothing else on because it made me feel fancy and womanly and queenlike. Nobody stopped me. My hair was very short, so when I think back I realize I must have looked more like the Little Prince than a princess as I paraded around the house with our two pet pugs, Mugsy and Sushi, as escorts. I was allowed to do these things because as long as I wasn't actually in danger, there were no rules. I took my mother's ashtrays and used them as plates for my doll tea parties. All of her things were nicer than mine—my things were made of plastic, hers were made of porcelain. All little girls like to have fancy things that belong to their mothers, and I was no exception. It is our right as daughters.

* * *

One of the other times they let my mother come home, I was on the staircase with my knees between the balusters and she was in the kitchen wearing her swooshy sweat suit like always, this time in turquoise. She was screaming at the top of her lungs about I don't know what, I just remember that she looked like a demon in the body of a giant Barbie doll with the kind of bird's-nest hair your Barbie gets when you brush it too much. She was yelling at my dad who was on the other side of the doorway just out of sight. He never yelled back, not once. I remember that more than feeling scared, I was curious. How could someone yell so loudly and channel so much anger? Each shout built momentum like a snowball that keeps gathering more of itself as it rolls downhill and nothing can stop the avalanche it becomes. She was interesting to me like the movie *Fantasia* is interesting.

It just keeps building with no clear narrative or rules. Colorful, cacophony mommy, so helpless and so powerful.

I was hungry and wanted cereal but I didn't dare go down there to the screaming zone. So I just stared at my mother from my staircase perch. I was frustrated that I couldn't exert my childlike urges when she was around. When a little kid is hungry it is her right to demand attention until the hunger is solved. But with my mom around, I had to be a quiet pair of eyes with no needs. Most young kids are only concerned with how the world makes *them* feel, but I saw the world as a place I needed to navigate in a more thoughtful way. To me, it felt more sad than unfair. Because as I watched my mom in that moment, I realized, *she could not handle her shit*. I felt, for the first time in my life, sad for another human being. And when you feel sad for someone it's very hard to resent them, even if they're hurting you. But it's also impossible to admire and look up to someone you feel sorry for.

My dad taught me to view my mom with compassion. He explained that she wasn't the boss of herself. I knew that also meant that she was not the boss of me. How could she be? A role model is supposed to be someone who knows more than you, someone who is a step *beyond where you are*. My mother was not a step beyond. She was not anywhere in my vicinity. Even though I was curious about what it would feel like to receive love and attention and affection and guidance from her, at the same time, I knew that she wasn't going to be able to do that for me. Nor was she someone to imitate. I was still desperately curious about her, but I knew it was best not to get too close. And this made me feel fundamentally different from other little girls and their moms, orbiting each other like a planet and its moon as they walked down the bike path behind my house to feed the ducks. I saw then that I was going to have to be my own planet, or maybe an asteroid floating free.

* * *

The third memory of my mother is violent and terrifying and I try not to think of it very often. It must have happened sometime after we shared the cigarette. I remember going into my parents' room unannounced, as kids often do. The bedroom light was off but the bathroom light was on. My parents' bathroom had those round bulbs that make you look like a movie star and the light spilled out into the dark bedroom, beckoning me to investigate. I crept forward . . . and there, in the mirror above the sink, I saw my mother glamorously illuminated. She was making a back-and-forth motion with one arm and she was very focused, with her attention completely centered on what she was doing, as though she were a concert violinist playing a slow, passionate solo underneath a spotlight. It was almost beautiful. But I tiptoed closer and saw that she wasn't holding a delicate violin bow; she was gripping a mean-looking metal saw with a wooden handle and a long triangular blade with big rusty teeth and raking it back and forth on her own body. There was a gaping bloody gash where her arm met her shoulder and I could see her muscles and bones, pulpy and dark, as she sawed. She cut through her own flesh as steadily as if she were carving a giant undercooked pot roast. Except she wasn't carving a pot roast, she was sawing off her own arm. This was and still is the most violent and sad thing I have ever seen. The older I get, the sadder this memory makes me—not for me, but for her.

I knew that what I was seeing wasn't right. My mom wasn't showing any signs of pain, which was confusing to me because I knew that blood meant *pain*. I spent a lot of time playing outside and I'd taken my share of bad falls. When you bled, it meant you were hurt and then you cried. So why wasn't my mom crying? I stood motionless, processing. I couldn't look away.

Then she turned around and saw me. She caught me catching her. Who was in bigger trouble? I knew I was seeing something I shouldn't and I wondered what kind of trouble I would be in for walking in on this. She stopped sawing for a moment but she didn't seem upset that I was there. She didn't even seem surprised. I can't remember *ever* seeing her act surprised, which is a quality I now associate with a sane person—the capacity for surprise. My mom and I have the same thick eyebrows and hers were not curved up in astonishment, angled down in anger, or drooping sideways with sadness. They were completely flat.

"What are you doing?" I asked. I knew what she was doing, but I also didn't know what she was *doing*.

"Don't tell your father," she replied, holding a flat stare for a beat before returning to her task.

The gears in my head whirred. My mother gave me an order, but even as a four-and-a-half-year-old, my instincts told me this was not right. So I ran. I used my legs intentionally and purposefully for the very first time to save my mom's life. I ran down the hall and found my dad. What's strange is that I cannot remember what happened after that, not even the moment I found my dad. I only know I was a big fat tattletale and she didn't die that day so I must have found him in time. My dad has always been there when I needed him.

After she was taken to the hospital, I tried to make sense of what I had seen. My dad never talked to me about this experience, maybe hoping it would fade on its own like a bruise, but it didn't fade and we never talked about it. The only point of reference I had was from Saturday-morning cartoons. There is a Looney Tunes trope where Bugs Bunny or Yosemite Sam or the Big Bad Wolf will use a saw—the same kind of wood-handled, triangular saw my mom used—to sabotage another character in some mischievous way. I remember the saw made an appearance at least once in every episode. So when I recognized the same cartoon saw in my mom's hand, my four-year-old mind experienced a reality warp where the line between the cartoon world and the real world was shattered. If things that happen in the cartoon world can happen in real life, I reasoned, then *anything is possible*. I understood that of course cartoons were not real, but my mind stretched in both directions like Silly Putty: If the most unimaginably *terrible* things are possible, like your mother sawing her arm off in front of you, then the most magically *good* things must also be possible, like, well, *anything*. That day, I saved her life, but I also had to save my own. I chose optimism. Life never serves you the lessons you need in the way you might imagine you'd receive them, but the lessons are nonetheless there, even if they are embedded in blood.

* * *

I have one good memory of my mother that I hold on to. It begins and ends in about four seconds, like a dream you try to keep when you first wake up but inevitably slips away as the day sets in. In the memory, I'm on the path that leads from our house to the lagoon where kids feed the ducks and I am riding my two-wheeler bike for the first time. As I pedal, I look back over my shoulder and I see my mother standing in the doorframe of our house watching me. She is actually *watching me*! She wears a sweat suit like always and she's smoking a cigarette, but she is *paying attention to me*. The feeling of being watched is the next best thing to being touched. It's like sunlight on your skin, as though the person watching you is giving you some part of themselves by way of their eyes.

The memory stops when I look back and see her. I don't really know what happened after that moment—I don't know if I fell down, or if she turned and went back inside, or if I just rode away. What is important is the memory of her eyes on me. My dad later confirmed that my mother did indeed teach me how to ride a bike, so now in my mind I've added a part at the beginning where she pushes me in a grand send-off, hands hovering attentively over my shoulders to catch me if I fall. And even though I don't know if that part is true, I've imagined it so many times that it *feels* true.

I often imagine things into existence until I don't know the difference between what is real and what isn't, what doesn't exist and what *could* exist if I believe it hard enough. I've visualized so many wonderful things into reality for myself. Becoming an Olympian took an extraordinary amount of hard work, but all it started with my belief that it could be true. Imagination, at the very least, brings us joy; at the very most, it empowers us to suspend disbelief and chase the impossible. Imagining things into existence is a superpower. The only sad part is that there will always be one thing I can never imagine into existence: having my mom back. But anything else is fair game.

* * *

One day my mother finally got away and did the thing she was trying to do. It was the middle of the night and we were all asleep. We've always been heavy sleepers in my family. But my dad woke up and realized she was gone, and when he searched the house he found a knife and blood on the floor of the downstairs bathroom. He would have probably been able to trace the blood to her body had it not been pouring rain outside. He called the security guards that patrolled our island city and they found her among the trees along the lagoon's edge, right where everyone feeds the ducks, next to the path where she taught me to ride my bike.

What gets me the most is that after she fatally cut herself, my mother made one last decision: She used her remaining strength to get out of the house where we were all asleep and go someplace to die where we wouldn't find her body. This small fact makes all the difference in the world. I like to believe that even though she was gripped by anguish so severe that she wanted to die, her final thoughts were of protecting my dad, my brother, and me. For my mother, this gesture was as thoughtful as she could have been. It makes me so grateful and also so sad. I hold on to this thoughtfulness as tightly as I would have held on to her if I could.

* * *

Did you ever realize *funeral* has the word *fun* in it? The cemetery where we buried my mom was surrounded by these irresistible hills and I remember my brother, Louis, and I ran up and down the grassy slopes having a grand time. There were even ducks nearby, like the lagoon in our neighborhood. But here there were no moms and daughters out for strolls, just crying people. I wore a pretty dress that got very dirty and a single shiny earring. Before the funeral I had begged my dad to take me to get my ears pierced, but after one ear I decided it hurt too much and ran out of the store before they could finish the job.

The congregation around my mother's grave was the largest group of people I'd ever seen gathered on account of one person. Everyone was dressed in fancy clothes like we were all going to see *The Nutcracker*. But instead of watching dancers, it felt like everyone was watching me. The adults looked at me like I was a perfectly good bag of popcorn that had been forgotten in the microwave and burned to a crisp. I imagine they were thinking, *This poor girl. How will she ever turn out okay? She doesn't even have both ears pierced!*

After she died, there were many more people suddenly involved in our life. Before she died, it was easier to keep her condition quiet. Back then mental illness wasn't handled openly with flowers and get-well cards like there might have been if she had been sick with cancer. My mother's depression was easy to keep out of sight. Her side of the family was out of the picture, both before and after her death—when she was living they refused to acknowledge she was sick, and when she died nobody from her family even came to the funeral, except for her father—and so my dad was left on his own throughout my mom's illness.

But after she died my family's secrets became public knowledge to everyone but me. I knew my mom had been unwell but I didn't learn the exact details of her death until years later. At the time, I thought she died from smoking cigarettes. Nobody corrected my assumption.

There was a flock of ladies who descended upon our house after the funeral. I still don't know who they were or how they knew us. I've never asked my dad, and for years if any woman looked at me for a second too long, I'd wonder if she had been one of them. They were all dressed up and they drank wine and I thought we were having a party. But it wasn't a party—it was a purging. They went through our house and stuffed everything that belonged to my mother in trash bags to be given away. These women were not just throwing my mother's things away—they were trying to throw *her* away, to erase her. When I realized what was occurring, I became a thief. I secretly grabbed all that my little hands could carry, which only amounted to her fur coat, a pair of Gucci shoes, and one photo album. We also had to give away our two adorable pugs, Mugsy and Sushi, because they had been my mom's dogs. My dad was working, and my brother and I were too young to be responsible for them. I wish I had been able to keep more of her clothes and other heirlooms, but I was denied this inheritance. I still wonder sometimes where my mom's clothes ended up and who in the world is wearing them.

The photo album I took dated back to my mother's teenage years and includes many pictures of her with young men who are most definitely *not* my dad. She looked like a young Elizabeth Taylor. Some of the pictures had love notes written on the back. I would have liked to have more pictures of her with my family, but I also enjoyed daydreaming about what she was like in high school. I imagined what kind of teenager she was and if I would be like her when I was that age. She was pretty, and it seemed like lots of people liked her. Most of all, it seemed like she liked herself. I kept the photo album hidden in my closet along with her Gucci shoes, which seemed more like Christmas tree ornaments than shoes because her feet were so small. Her fur coat became my favorite article of clothing. I loved how it felt grand, worn, pre-loved. To this day, I never feel guilty about spending money on vintage clothes. I feel I deserve to have certain old things I'll never be given by my mom.

Recently, I discovered that the photo album and the coat and the shoes aren't the only things I inherited from my mother. I learned on an episode of the podcast *Radiolab* that all humans carry around a unique set of microbes that live on our skin, which "colonize" us as we pass through the birth canal. The microbes literally jump from our mother's uterus and vagina and set up shop on our newborn skin. Regardless of where we move around the world or the countless interactions we have throughout our life, our skin microbes will always be descendants from the original microbes we inherited from our mothers at birth.

I was devastated when I first learned this fact. Knowing that I literally carry my mother with me made me feel like I was infected with some dark thing. But then I came to feel comforted by this inheritance. What about those times in summer camp when everyone got sick but me? Or the intimate moments when boys tell me I smell nice even when I'm sweaty? It must have been her microbes. I look at how far I've come and I see that my mother's microbes have been my invisible teammates. I understand that even if her illness prevented her from raising me, part of her has been with me all along.

All dead people should know this: They're going to matter, even if they think they won't and even if they don't want to. I understand now that toward the end, my mother was so sick that she didn't want to be part of this world any longer. She thought she could fade away. But her absence meant as much to me as her presence would have.

Maybe my mom thought that she was being kind to me by leaving—that because she was gone I wouldn't have to deal with having a crazy mother. But by leaving the way she did, my mother actually burdened me with the task that would come to define my young adult life: to grow up without her.

if an oyster can turn sand into pearls

i can turn myself into anything

GIRL SCOUTS

My brother taught me to pee standing up. That's how people pee, duh. He'd also dress me up in my dad's work suits and make me sit on the toilet with a newspaper in my hands and wait for my dad to come home. He would tell me, "See, this is how he does it." One time my dad was late coming home and I waited for an hour on the toilet reading an article I couldn't understand. My dad came home and found me, and that was when he decided I needed to be around more women.

My dad has always liked to live within what might be considered traditional parameters. He orders *classic* breakfasts like waffles, western omelets, and eggs Benedict. He introduced me to *classic* sports like baseball, soccer, basketball, and track. He still signs my presents "From Santa." So naturally, when he sought out female mentorship for me, he turned to the most classically female environment available: the Girl Scouts.

I was six years old when he first signed me up, and being at Girl Scout meetings felt like stepping through a kaleidoscope peephole into a glittery female world that both intimidated and fascinated me. Up until that point, I had only really been surrounded by men and animals: my dad, my brother, our pugs,

and our cats. But my weekly Girl Scout meetings were the do-
main of *the mom*. The troop leaders were all moms and they'd
lead us scouts in weekly meetings where we'd learn how to sew,
do crafts, and cook pancakes on upside-down Folgers coffee tins
with tea candles underneath. I felt more comfortable being the
only girl at Boy Scouts than being surrounded by girls at Girl
Scouts. (I know this because I went to multiple Boy Scout meetings and trips when it was my dad's turn to chaperone my
brother's troop and he could not leave me home alone.) At Girl
Scout meetings I felt the constant presence of a mom hovering
over me in a way that was deeply unfamiliar. I had never felt a
woman's chest accidentally brush against me before. Charm
necklaces dangled onto my shoulder like fairies and perfume
cascaded over me as the mom-leaders helped stitch the crotch
together on my pair of homemade pajamas. Other girls weren't
distracted by the approach of a mom-leader and could keep
working on their crafts despite being watched by mom-eyes, but
not me. I was always taken aback when one of them turned her
attention to me, and I couldn't focus on anything else.

I was confronted by new female things, like cheeks dusted
with noticeable veils of face powder, eyes outlined in eyeliner,
exposed bra lines, soft skin, manicured toes, dyed hair. I also
absorbed the way they talked, the way they disciplined, the way
they loved. It was intellectually instructional but emotionally
painful. It felt like touching hot candle wax, where you want to
do it and still keep doing it even though it hurts. These moms
were not like my mom at all. My mom, when she was home,
was liable to explode into a fit of rage at any moment. She was
not to be approached. I knew she would never harm me physically, but when she'd yell at the toaster in the kitchen because

she thought it was talking to her, my instincts told me to keep my guard up.

At first I was wary and even afraid of these Girl Scout mom-leaders. It was overwhelming and strange to be around them, and I didn't like when they paid too much attention to me, as if to overcompensate for the things they knew I was missing at home. They projected a *lack* onto me that I still cannot fully understand. It's a lack that other people feel on my behalf. When I was a kid these looks felt like a challenge or a puzzle; I didn't know exactly what I was missing, but *they did*.

When the mom-leaders spoke to me, I fumbled in my inter-actions with them. I didn't know how to handle being around mothers like this. I didn't know the right way to handle being touched—I have no memories of my mom ever touching me, and my dad only touched me when he was showing me how to play sports or giving me an occasional hug. I didn't know how to be disciplined by or properly receive a talking-to from a woman; I didn't know how to take a compliment or otherwise respond to *being mothered*. But I didn't want them to think I didn't know how. I tried to respond the way I felt you were sup-posed to because I wanted them to think I understood my role in this equation. I wanted to pass whatever aptitude test they were giving me, not be the poor little girl with the dead mom.

Within the incubator of my own home, I never felt *watched* like I did at Girl Scouts. In my recollection, nobody in my house watched me. My dad or an au pair was always around in case I got hurt, but I was never watched in the literal sense of the word. Girl Scout moms were constantly in a state of anticipation of one of us needing help—the kind of help their mom-intuition told them we needed without us asking for it. Before I even had the chance to accidentally overfill my Folgers tin with pancake batter, an eager mom would swoop in and save the day: "This is how much pancake batter to use, dear." This was the land of dears, honeys, sweeties, and pumpkins. I will never forget the time I was voraciously sucking on a lemon wedge and one of the moms reached over from behind my back and snatched it away, telling me my teeth would rot if I ate raw lemons. I was hurt and insulted: I had packed those lemon wedges myself and even sprinkled them with sugar—how many of the other scouts had prepared their own snacks? None, that's how many. I felt suffocated by the unsolicited commentary.

Is it such a big deal for a kid to eat raw lemons or spill pancake batter? I would have preferred to learn the hard way. But I'm sure that even if my Folgers tin *did* overflow, one of the moms would have materialized with a damp paper towel to scoop up all the raw batter before I could eat it, as I would have done if left to my own devices. Being surrounded by these moms made me feel less capable. I didn't like being watched so closely, so suddenly, so constantly.

My mom never watched me like these moms did. In our house, my mom was the one who needed to be observed and helped, not me. Most times when my mother and I were actually in the same space, which in itself was rare, she seemed either to not realize I was there or to just not care. In the rare moments when my mom did look at me, she usually looked *through* me. We were cohabitants of the space and she was going to keep being her while I kept being me. This was our understanding. And even though I *did* want a mom, a real mom, I also liked the freedom I had. I was able to try things like scooping generous handfuls of wet dog food into my mouth or killing dozens of backyard slugs. How do you understand the gravity and guilt of killing slugs you collected in a shoebox and sprinkled with salt if you are stopped mid-mission by someone who already knows better?

All the most important lessons in life we have to learn for ourselves. The sooner we realize this the better. How are you supposed to learn anything if you aren't allowed to try things? How do you know what's on the other side of a cliff if you're never allowed close enough to peek over the edge? In a way, my mom and I were *both* allowed to be reckless around each other. She made me feel capable for reasons I still can't fully explain or justify. I don't mean to glorify her illness, I'm just saying that someone as tortured inside her own head as my mother was doesn't have the capacity to insert themselves into someone else's, for better and for worse. For better because when I was around her I had the unusual freedom to push the boundaries of my curiosity, and for worse because I knew if I asked her for help I wouldn't get it.

* * *

My dad grew up abroad, in Saudi Arabia, part of a Greek American family working in the oil industry, and he was independent from a very young age. American school in Saudi Arabia stopped after middle school, so he went to an all-boys boarding school in New Jersey for high school and then to Brown University. He went alone—even though he was close to his parents, they never traveled to the States to visit him and they did not come to his graduations. My dad found his way just as I had to find my way, and it never occurred to him to hover

over me like the Girl Scout moms did. It simply wasn't in his parenting vocabulary.

My friends' parents, on the other hand, had attention to spare. I learned this from countless playdates at their houses where their moms were not only present but *active participants*, enhancing the playdate with craft projects and snacks. I rarely had friends over because my dad worked so much, and even when he was home I never liked other people seeing the waist-high mountains of newspapers that covered the majority of our floor, or the general lack of rules and supervision at our house. My friends loved it because my house felt like a mystical playland with vague parental authority on the periphery—the polar opposite of their regimented existences of plastic sippy cups and time-outs. To my friends, my house symbolized freedom. To me, my friends' houses symbolized a curated life that I both haughtily reviled and desperately craved.

I do believe there's a healthy spectrum of parental attention that exists, with my dad closer to one end of the spectrum and a helicopter parent on the opposite end. But here's the thing: On the helicopter side of the spectrum, at its very worst, a parent's personal ego can become wrapped up in his or her kid's life. They see their kid as a reflection of themselves and they can't bear to let the kid out of their grip.

As an adult, I so often notice parents telling their kids that their hair looks so good this way or that, or how they might try pushing their nail cuticles down just a tad, or a million other small things that seem like no big deal but are actually just one of a million small ways to make a kid feel ever so much more under their parent's thumb. Parents aren't meant to protect their kids from failure or heartbreak or being ugly—those things are all a natural part of growing up and figuring things out. I get that it can be hard for parents to let go in this way and watch their kid flounder. It's not a very pretty sight. Maybe for a parent, the hardest thing to do is to let their kid fail. But I believe that reducing a child's pain to nothing is far worse.

I see often this dynamic at play in the running world. In Mammoth Lakes, my high-altitude training camp, there's a father-son duo that I see at the gym. The dad stalks behind his high-school-aged son, pushing him to do one more rep, and the kid has a permanent scowl on his face. I'm sure the dad feels very proud of his son. And who knows what the son feels, probably some mixture of pressure and pride. I'm sure the son is a very fast runner. But this sort of dynamic is rarely sustainable. If a kid only knows how to thrive under the guiding hand of a parent, however eager and well-intentioned the parent is, then they might be good at running in high school and get recruited to a top running college—but when they get there and are suddenly on their own, their whole world implodes. I personally witnessed this type of saga unfold numerous times during my NCAA career. There's a huge difference between opening doors for your kid and pushing them through.

My dad never told me to go to bed early, never wrote one of my essays for me, and never sat me down and told me not to drink. He didn't necessarily know that my friends and I were sneaking into Cal college parties or having bonfires on Ocean Beach, but he made sure I always had a safe way to get around and a safe place to stay. It was up to me to bounce within those barriers. I know my dad would have stepped in more forcefully had he seen me being unsafe or trending in a dangerous direction, but since I wasn't, my decisions were up to me. He would have been fine if I got B's in school—I was the one who wanted all A's. He would have been fine if I stopped playing sports forever—I was the one who committed to running competitively in college. I know that if I had felt even a drop of pressure from my dad when I stopped running my junior year of high school and played soccer instead, I might have done something that wasn't in my best long-term interest. I might have burned out as a runner and never become an Olympian. It's not that my dad didn't care about running. If I'd dropped out of running and spent my time doing nothing, he would have intervened. But when I *did* stop running partway through high school and focused on soccer instead, he saw I was happier on the soccer field and left it at that. He didn't care that I had more competitive potential as a runner—he just cared that I was busy and safe. Maybe he knew that, like my mom, I was always hardest on myself. It wouldn't have helped to be pushed. He never pushed. He bent over backward to ensure that I had opportunities—in middle school my dad would drive me from soccer practice to softball practice to cross-country meets, shielding me with a towel as I changed from one uniform into the next—but when we got to the activity, he let me do my thing. Whether I won a race or crawled across the finish line (both have happened multiple times), we'd go out for late-night pizza all the same. Since my dad's ego never stood between me and my failures and successes, my failures and successes were entirely my own. I owned them, all of them.

For young Alexi, Girl Scouts was a weekly interruption to the life of independence I had at home with my dad and brother. I became self-conscious underneath the Scout moms' constant observation and I started questioning my every move. At the same time, I felt I was stronger and wiser than the other girls who had moms—how do you become confident and independent if you are constantly given a helping hand, even when you might not need it? I know I may be insulting every mom walking this earth and I'm sorry for that. But before moms ever helped me, they hurt me. Though I'm certain it was unintentional, they made me feel I was lacking something fundamental. They pushed too much, too soon.

* * *

One time I peed in my sleeping bag during a Girl Scout camping trip, and I concocted an elaborate story about how a raccoon had entered the old manor where we all bunked, crept into my sleeping bag, and peed. I then went on to explain how I heroically scared it away before it could pee in anyone else's sleeping bag—thereby justifying the presence of urine in only my sleeping bag. All the girls believed me, but the mom-leaders pulled me aside and told me they knew I was lying, and lying was *very bad*. My dad had to make the hour-long drive to the campsite to deliver a fresh sleeping bag, but he didn't have anything to say about my raccoon cover story. This lie didn't actually hurt anybody. My dad knew when to let me take care of myself in the ways I knew how.

I know the Girl Scout moms made sure to notify him about my big lie, and I could tell that they were disappointed he didn't discipline me. This made me very angry. I've always hated it when I can tell that my dad feels judged by other parents, however subtly. There are lots of things most parents do that my dad never did. I have never and probably never will share forks, cups, or plates with my dad. He'd rather order me my own hot chocolate than give me a sip of his. I have never had the nightmares cuddled out of me, either—he preferred to stand in my doorway and watch me fall asleep on my own.

But I knew that my dad loved me more than anything in the world, just in his own specific and intentional ways. Every night when he tucked me in he would say, without fail, "You know, you're a good kid, Lex. Did anyone ever tell you you're a good kid?" He repeated this ritual every single night, and I used to think he was crazy. But he was just parenting in the way he knew how. Hugs and cuddles weren't his way—his was a more nitty-gritty, showing-up-every-day kind of effort. I think he was telling me, and also himself, that yes, I was turning out okay. I was doing an all right job and he was doing an all right job. And if it had been done any other way, I wouldn't be who I am today. I've learned that it's not productive to wonder too much about what my life could have been like if things had been different. I once read that the chances of any person being born as themselves instead of as a different genetic combination is estimated to be the same as if two million people rolled a trillion-sided die and all got the same number. We are who we are. We are all little marvels.

My dad had to leave the campsite shortly after making the sleeping-bag delivery because there were NO BOYS ALLOWED. I was sad to see him go and stewed in my shame, thinking I was destined to forever feel out of place in this Girl Scout world. But then the sun went down and the moms built a campfire and we sang songs and ate s'mores and I felt a shift, as if the darkness and the flickering campfire allowed me to blend in with the other girls and forget the thing that made me different. Being one silhouette among many gathered around the campfire felt deeply *good*, like the gooey center of a roasted marshmallow. It was the first time I can remember when I didn't feel responsible for myself. I was a part of a crowd of little girls and sillies and I really appreciate that the moms let us kids *just be*. I finally allowed myself to fit in like one marshmallow among many.

Sometimes feeling *undifferentiated* is the nicest feeling in the world. Nobody looked at me like I needed special help. I felt included but not scrutinized. I let go of my anxiety, like when you don't realize you're clenching your jaw but then you open your mouth for a moment and, suddenly, you feel relief. At least for the moment, I stopped labeling myself as different. I licked my marshmallow fingers, touched the cool earth under my little butt, and felt, for the first time, like a kid.

I haven't officially quit the Girl Scouts. I think I may even still be a member on a list somewhere deep within my troop's archives. The troop moms will always hold a special place in my heart. I am sure I was as much a handful to them as they were to me. I want them to know it was worth the effort.

i admire pickles because there is no one moment
that makes a pickle

a pickle. it is a thing that happens over time.
pickles are patient.

A VERY BIG ALEXI

Because my dad had to work so much, he hired live-in au pairs who would stay with us for a year at a time when I was in elementary school. They were always between nineteen and twenty-two years old and female, which my dad felt was important. Some wore bras and some didn't, and they all smelled nice even without deodorant. They seemed to me to be a very specific kind of woman, the type who ate sweets whenever she wanted and said what was on her mind without thinking twice. They weren't afraid to touch my hair and wipe my face when I had smudgy chocolate streaks around my mouth. I ate the best chocolate growing up because all of it was from Europe, brought by the au pairs or sent to them in care packages from their homeland.

The visas these au pairs were on only let them stay with us for one year and not a day longer. This wasn't up to me, this was up to the government. The government doesn't care at all if you loved this au pair so much you wished she would stay forever, or if you hated that au pair so much that you wanted her to leave *right this instant*. I treated my au pairs like single-serving disposable mothers. I squeezed everything I could out of them. This was my right—they were there to be my surrogate moms. Some of them I hated. But the ones I loved, I really *loved*. I loved them in an unreasonable way that can only come from a place of extreme desperation, and an awareness that one day in the near future they would be gone. I loved them fiercely as if they were terminally ill, because to me what was the difference? As far as I was concerned, all of my au pairs had one year to live.

Each au pair taught me how to count to ten in her home language, so I can count to ten in about eight different Eastern European languages, and maybe more if I really try. One of the au pairs stole jewelry and money from us. Some of them crashed our family car and others stayed out way too late at night on this likely first-time trip to the United States. But my dad never got angry, and he never fired them before their one-year tenure was up because he must have judged that these infractions did not outweigh the benefits of having a female caretaker around my brother and me.

One year a new au pair arrived the day I got back from a weeklong campout with my fifth-grade class. It ended with everyone crying about how much they'd miss camp, but then the moment someone got off the bus they'd run straight to their mom to hug her so tight, and it was clear they'd instantly forgotten about their camp life and were now thrilled to come back to the comforts of home. I was the only one who didn't have a mom waiting at the bus stop, but I still decided to do like the other kids did. I ran to my new au pair—a complete stranger—and hugged her like she was someone I had known my whole life and had missed terribly during this week away from home. I remember actually watching other kids hugging their moms and taking mental notes, as if leaping into a woman's arms just the right way might make her feel like home and not a stranger. I was acutely aware that the woman I was hugging looked nothing like me, whereas everyone else looked at least a little bit like their mom, but I didn't mind: I was just happy to have a new woman in my life, even if it was only a gesture at the maternal figure that everyone else had. In a situation like mine you can't afford to be picky.

After our embrace, I learned my new au pair's name. She was Petra, from the Czech Republic.

* * *

Petra became my first real role model. She was the tallest woman I had ever seen, with short hair that was dyed auburn and broad shoulders. Her teeth were not perfect. She ate like a lumberjack and would carry me around under her arm like a bundle of firewood. She liked real maple syrup and couldn't stand processed food. She folded our clothes because it was part of her job but she played with my brother and me like it was her passion. Petra could make a game out of anything, like what she called "pulling back the cloud," which was when you use a spoon to pull the foam back on a cappuccino and pour a packet of sugar in and then let the cloud close again. I loved it.

Petra was calm but sharp. She asked what books I was reading and what they were about. She showed me how a woman can be confident and curious at the same time. Petra spoke to me like an adult, as if she were talking to a peer, or as if she were a high-end chef speaking to a distinguished diner: "And how is the macaroni and cheese tonight?" It proved that Petra was invested in me, however short our time together was.

Petra also coached my basketball team. She could take on a court of five opponents and win. She could jump, she could shoot, she could touch the rim—to me, Petra was unstoppable and infinite. She was the first female athlete I saw achieve something that I never imagined a person could do. By this time, I was a little Olympian in the making. I loved every sport I played, from basketball to softball to soccer to tennis. The only thing I liked more than playing was winning, because winning was a fact. I liked how winning felt, like it was something good I had in my control, something that couldn't be taken away from me.

At home I followed Petra around, copying the things she ate and did and said. I attached myself to Petra like a well-intentioned leech. She would drink exclusively out of our glass Coca-Cola cups and she wore plain white V-necked T-shirts that she made into tank tops, so I stole my dad's undershirts and cut the sleeves off to fashion them like Petra's. I know he wondered where his shirts went, but I never got in trouble. Petra used the phrase "This is suck" to describe things she didn't like, such as bad coffee, so I adopted it, too. "This is suck," I'd say about having to do my homework.

I also copied Petra's basketball warm-up routine. I felt much more capable when I imitated her than when I was being myself. She used to shoot hoops in our driveway every day, and I would sometimes watch her from the window—I'm fairly certain she could see my little face smashed against the glass, but she never said anything. I appreciated that she let me watch her without pointing it out. It can be embarrassing to admire someone so much, and I needed to be able to copy her without her acknowledging that I was copying her. By letting my observations and imitations pass unspoken, Petra gave me confidence while also preserving my dignity. This was a gift.

I finally confessed to Petra that I wanted to climb out of myself and literally *become her*. I was desperate; her year was almost up and she would be leaving soon. I loved being around her and I hated that I wouldn't be able to absorb her powers through osmosis forever. But I didn't have those words yet. I could only climb onto her lap while we were watching TV and confess: "Petra, I want to be you."

Petra turned the TV off and looked at me, really looked at me. I took in her auburn bowl cut and crooked teeth as if I were gazing upon a fairy-tale queen. "Don't be me," she said in her accented English. "Be a very big Alexi instead."

At first, this answer upset me. I was annoyed to be receiving advice that I needed rather than the kind that I wanted. I would have liked for Petra to tell me that yes, I could become her, and also that she'd stay and be my au pair forever. But that was not possible. Petra knew I needed to learn that it is useful to look up to people, but not to try and literally become them.

We should never want to become anyone else, because the greatest fulfillment we can ever get out of life is by becoming the best possible version of ourselves. To magically become someone else would be to skip the journey of becoming our ultimate thing, our *very big selves*. It might seem easier that way, but it isn't better. Petra was empowering me rather than sheltering me. She was wise to send me off like this, with honesty and integrity, even if it hurt.

When Petra left she sent us chocolates, like a distant relative might, but the fancy European chocolate didn't taste good to me. It was a reminder that I was going to have to grow up and be on my own. I hated that feeling, but I also knew I would be okay, just like Petra knew I would be. I think the reason why it hurt so badly when Petra left is that deep down I knew I could do it; I knew I had it in me to become *a very big Alexi*. I knew I could grow the invisible but real muscle called *confidence* all on my own. Petra opened the door to that realization, but I had to walk through it on my own.

Sometimes it hurts to know you can do it. It's an intimidating thing to realize because it means that the only person who can really define your growth and happiness is yourself. There is no shortcut to becoming your best self. The responsibility is on you.

headed to the moon

not now but soon

THE MENTOR BUFFET

I always appreciate when women I admire let me close to them. I never liked female mentorship when it was forced on me, as it was in Girl Scouts, but I *loved* it when I could seek it out on my own terms.

The first female mentors I felt drawn to were my best friends' moms. Until the day I left for college I had a stable of moms in my orbit, inviting me over for dinner or bringing me to nail salons or chaperoning me at concerts. I had a special relationship with these moms—if a friend and her mom were arguing about how we weren't allowed to leave the house to walk around our small city after dark, the mom would always turn to me, as if performing an aside in a play, and smile, shrug her shoulders, and say, "That's just how it is! I know, I know, I'm a mean old mom."

As a non-mommed kid, I could never be fully folded into the mother-daughter dynamic. I existed somewhere outside of that food chain. I was not a daughter with a mother of her own waiting at home (moms seem to generally know not to encroach on each other's territory) nor was I an adult peer. I was an exciting project. This was very attractive to moms, and it was a role I was glad to fill—because it came with benefits. I was allowed to be present with friends and their moms in moments when an outsider might not normally be included, like going to the pool and not being asked to leave the bathroom stall when it was the mom's turn to change. This is how I was introduced to the adult vagina. I remember all the mom-vaginas I ever saw because it felt like seeing a sea otter in San Francisco Bay: not impossible but definitely not an everyday occurrence. It was thrilling to catch a glimpse of what I might expect from my own body one day. This wasn't something I could ask of anyone. It had to be offered. I am very grateful for the moms who performed subtle acts of unveiling like this for me.

I also absorbed tremendous amounts of knowledge and wisdom from women I didn't know at all, whom I'd observe in brief moments throughout my everyday life: at the grocery store, or in a dentist's waiting room, or in a public restroom while the lady next to me examined her face in the mirror. I think about this now whenever I catch a little girl staring at me in a public bathroom or in line at the store or across an airport terminal waiting area. I wonder how much of an impact I might be making without my knowing it. As a child, I was a highly adept observer, logging every small detail in just a few seconds. With each new tidbit of womanly knowledge I gleaned, the world of the feminine widened a bit.

In middle school my friend Kati's mom often invited me over for dinner after school because she knew my dad worked late, and by then I was too old for au pairs but too young to be responsible for meals every night after school, practice, and homework. I probably ate dinner with Kati's family twice a week. Two family dinners per week is an above-average amount to be eating at your friend's house, but it was either go to Kati's where there was a thoughtfully prepared meal or be at home alone. My dad often worked well past the dinner hour and I'd be left to cook for myself. I knew he was doing the best he could, and he cooked great meals when he was able, but I have always loved good food and I've never been too proud to seek it out. I think Kati's mom invited me over not just for my own well-being but also because I genuinely loved the food she fed me and wasn't shy about expressing my gratitude. With each dish she placed before me, my excitement and awe were palpable. I would ask her, "What *is* this? How did you make this?" Every week she prepared things I'd never heard of before—osso buco, paella, and other dishes that perhaps were ordinary to her but that I thought were magnificent. She was always more than willing to take the time to answer my questions, like how often she went grocery shopping and how long to boil oatmeal and whether butter should be kept in the fridge or not. I learned that having genuine curiosity and gratitude was the best way to start a conversation with someone I hoped to learn something from.

I'd always ask Kati if we could do our homework at the kitchen table instead of upstairs in her bedroom. The view and the smells in the kitchen were wonderfully distracting, and I think Kati's mom knew I was watching her. I felt reassured by her presence. I pretended she was cooking especially for me as she layered lasagna and peeled cucumbers, and this made me feel loved in a way that I craved as much as I craved that lasagna. I imagined she laid the pasta sheets down atop the tomato sauce in the same way that she tucked her kids into bed at night. Why focus on algebra, which has been around forever and isn't going anywhere, when you can absorb something much more fleeting and rare like the sight of a mom making your dinner? I was prepped from very early in life to understand that some things last and some things do not. I always got seconds and thirds at Kati's house and I even took home leftovers. All I wanted to do was absorb more of that lasagna and more of that mom.

I asked Kati's mom to help me understand how I could become a good cook like her. Kati didn't need this knowledge yet, but I needed it now, since I was cooking dinner for myself a couple of times a week. I needed to understand how to love myself like Kati's mom loved her family. Food is a good way to show love to yourself. The meal I am most proud of was from a recipe Kati's mom shared with me. It is a beef pot roast that cooks itself during the day while you're not even home to watch it. Here is how you make it: Place a whole pot roast in the oven in the morning before school with onions and carrots and any spices you like, and then surround it with ice so that it keeps cool throughout the day. Then set the oven timer to turn on around the time that you finish school and the meal cooks while you're at soccer practice. The best feeling in the world is when you get back from soccer that evening and dinner is ready! I was so proud the first time I made that pot roast and arrived home to find my perfect treasure in the oven after a full day of anticipation. As I ate, I decided that I *liked* asking moms for advice and that I'd do it more often. In high school, I asked Kati's mom to help me sew my sophomore Winter Ball dress out of found fabric. She said yes without hesitation. It didn't feel dumb to ask for help, and in fact, I learned that it felt better to ask for help than to wait until someone noticed I needed it.

Asking for help is a superpower anyone can have but only

some people use. It is brave to ask for help. Asking for help is the first step toward finding a mentor. Mentors can help us change our lives if we let them.

* * *

When I went to college, I was drawn to confident women who were older and more experienced than me, women I admired and wanted to emulate. I had already developed the muscle that knows how to seek out mentors, so it was natural for me to transition from getting advice from my friends' moms to seeking out guidance from my female professors.

I attached myself to one professor in particular, Cynthia Huntington, who was my honors poetry thesis adviser in my senior year. The first thing I asked her was what I needed to do to become a better writer. From my experiences with friends' moms, I had learned that the best way to get a potential mentor to take you under her wing is to ask for advice and to be specific with your questions, and also to approach the conversation with an air of gratitude and genuine curiosity.

Cynthia told me, quite plainly, that I needed to read a lot more and write a lot more. I loved words, and I needed to consume and create a lot more of them. She taught me how to make writing my craft, just like running was, which meant it would take focus and time and dedication. Writing, like running, isn't an innate skill that we're born with—it's a discipline we can learn and develop. Cynthia told me that if I wrote fifteen poems in a day and just one of them was good, then it was a productive day. She recommended that I write in three- to six-hour chunks of uninterrupted time, not just half an hour here and there. She taught me how to commit to something challenging with assurance. I wanted to be a good writer—but more than that, I wanted to be like Cynthia. She carried herself with confidence. She watched people with curiosity but never jealousy. She liked herself. She made me believe I had control over my own destiny. If I could work toward becoming a better writer by becoming a student of writing, then I could also become the best me by becoming a student of myself.

Cynthia invited me to her house more than once, but the most memorable time was on my twenty-first birthday. I never turned down her invitations and I never said no to a home-cooked meal. She lived forty-five minutes from campus, deep in the woods of Vermont. I didn't have a car, so she decided that this dinner would be a sleepover. When I was younger I imagined that college would be like this—invitations to professors' homes and dinner parties—and I was so surprised to see it actually unfolding. I often feel like this when something special happens. At first I wonder how and why this special thing is happening, then, as I have learned, the answer is because I am a lucky person *and* I try to be the kind of person lucky things happen to. You have to believe you are deserving of good surprises in life. You set yourself up for it. You walk with your eyes open enough to catch the eye of the person who will invite you in. Maybe they won't *but maybe they will*. Luck can be cultivated.

Cynthia lived alone with her big dog, Sugar, a white husky whom she sometimes brought to class. Cynthia and Sugar would walk in the Vermont woods every morning while Cynthia foraged for wild mushrooms. For my birthday dinner we ate steak with mushrooms cooked in bacon fat. Sugar sat under the table and gnawed on the extra fat. Cynthia's floors were hardwood painted poppy blue. I'd never seen anyone paint color over hardwood floors before. She told me that the plain wood bored her.

At the time, I was Cynthia's most devoted poetry student and I was planning on pursuing a graduate degree in poetry. I had recently gotten the news that I had been awarded a full scholarship to three of the top MFA programs in the country, a dream come true for any aspiring poet. At the same time, I was also in touch with coaches from the University of Oregon, who were offering me a spot on their legendary cross-country team to run as a fifth-year super-senior. This offer was by no means a guarantee of an Olympic future, but it was definitely an opportunity to contribute to an NCAA championship-winning team and also explore where my running could take me—many great pro runners had come out of the UO program. I asked Cynthia for advice about which path I should take. Without missing a beat, she looked straight at me and told me I should use my body as best I can while it's still at my disposal.

I was in shock. I pushed back—surely, she couldn't be serious? I expected a creative mentor to nudge me toward the arts. But instead, Cynthia smiled and said, "Alexi, I think you should go all in and pursue running. You can write the rest of your life." When she smiles, it is in a way that makes you realize how little you truly know about her. She was battling the onset of MS, rendering her whole body very frail. You could tell when you looked at her that she'd led a wild life, and now her body, which had done so much *living*, was trying and failing to stand its ground against this disease. I felt sad for how imbalanced the picture was: me all potential at the beginning of my adult journey, she nearing the end of hers.

So when Cynthia advised me to accept UO's offer, I listened.

This conversation was about more than what classes I might take or what kind of boy I might date; we were making decisions about my future. And I could feel that she was giving me advice from a place of deep, true understanding. She knew better than I did not only that this athletic opportunity was rare and fleeting but also that it would complement my creative career. Even if they seem totally unrelated, becoming great in one discipline will always help in another. It is a gift to receive advice from someone who is fully grounded in themselves like this, and it was Cynthia's wisdom that gave me the courage to turn down my MFA scholarships and commit to an uncertain path toward the Olympics. For dessert Cynthia made me a birthday cake topped with a generous shelf of buttercream frosting. It was the best cake I've ever tasted because I knew she had made it just for me. I haven't had many homemade birthday cakes, so this meant a lot.

For breakfast we ate bacon and eggs cooked in bacon fat. I drank coffee from one of Cynthia's mugs, which was my favorite shade of matte red, and she told me to keep it. When I got back to campus, the sleepover felt like one of those experiences that must have happened to someone else. But I know it happened because I still have Cynthia's mug to prove it. It is my writing mug.

I realize that the stories in this chapter revolve around food, sewing, and beauty—but it was never the actual act of baking a cake or cooking a meal or sewing a dress that affected me, it was the *confidence* these women brought to their actions, confidence that was so strong and deep that I couldn't help but absorb some of it myself.

* * *

A good mentor is a living example of the type of person you'd like to be, and you can learn from them simply by being in their vicinity and paying attention. And the older I got, the more my hunger for mentors grew. I was always on the lookout.

The summer after college, I spent several weeks in Provincetown, Massachusetts, with my friend Abbey's aunt Mary and Mary's partner, Marion. Mary is a clothing designer and Marion is a painter and they let me fold in with their life. They woke me up at six o'clock and took me swimming naked in the ocean where we'd see famous writers standing on their decks writing their first pages of the day. Marion and Auntie Mary were in their sixties and had the vibrancy of teenagers. I felt lucky to be allowed into their space and I was happy to make their routines my own. I sat at their kitchen table like a kid after school, eating blueberries and listening to them talk about their artist life and their sugarless diet and their outdoor shower. They wanted to hear about my silly little movie, *Tracktown*, which at the time was just an idea. But the way they asked me about it made it seem like it *could* be real, like my idea wasn't silly and that I should take myself seriously. They never told me this directly—they didn't have to.

When I moved to Eugene, Oregon, to start my year at UO, I continued to consciously put myself in spaces with people I admired. To me, it was more important to be around the right people than anything else. During my time in Oregon I soaked up everything I could from my teammates, coaches, and the environment of a world-class athletic school. I was nervous to be competing in such a serious environment, which felt like a different world than Dartmouth running, but then before the NCAA Cross Country Championships in the fall the team captain pulled me aside and told me that *I could do it*. I ran an incredible race and we won that championship. I learned that I thrive when I'm around people who believe in themselves and in me.

After my fifth year at UO, I began life as an Olympic hopeful. I often took extended training trips to Mammoth Lakes, California, just to be closer to my biggest athletic role model, Deena Kastor, an Olympic bronze medalist and the American record holder for the marathon. I had always admired Deena from afar, but when she and her husband, Andrew, invited me to visit and train with the Mammoth Track Club, their training group, I leapt at the opportunity. When a woman you admire that much gives you the chance to get close to her, you take it.

I got nervous for every single long run and workout that I did with Deena, and there was one particular two-hour run that felt especially daunting. It was the longest run I'd ever done, and a long run is a hard thing to fake. The distance and pace were ambitious, but I didn't want to drop out early; I wanted to be alongside Deena for as long as possible. Sure enough, about an hour and a half into the run, I sensed the hurt coming on. My legs felt like two cylinders of canned cranberry sauce, splatting just a bit more with each step. If I had been alone, I would have slowed down. But that wasn't an option here. So I shifted my attention away from my own pain and instead focused on Deena. Specifically, I focused on her breath, which was calm compared to mine. I pretended she was breathing for both of us. She sensed my pain and distracted me by pointing out a passing hawk and trying to guess where it came from and where it was heading. I held on to our pace for the sake of hearing the rest of Deena's hawk fable. No one had told me spontaneous stories like this when I was a child, and I relished it deep in the youngest place in my heart.

Deena made me feel like a more capable athlete and she also made me feel like a more capable person. She pushed me from a place of magnanimous love. To be pushed by someone who truly believes in you is a huge gift. It is like they're pushing you and pulling you at the same time. It is a love that comes from a place of wanting you to be there with them.

* * *

It is not always easy to put yourself in the same spaces as the mentors you look up to. Sometimes I will go through Herculean efforts to put myself near a particularly tantalizing mentor. Take Rachel Dratch, who played my mother in my first movie, *Tracktown*. Rachel and I both went to Dartmouth and were even in the same college improv group, years apart. I also studied comedy at Second City just like she did. Despite these connections, Rachel was not immediately accessible to me. I had met her once, when she came to do a book signing at the Dartmouth bookstore, but I was among a crowd of other students who were also eager to meet her.

When my now-husband, Jeremy Teicher, and I wrote *Tracktown*, we wrote a role for Rachel with the hope that we might be able to ask her to consider being in our movie. We were able to get a copy of the script to Rachel through a connection in the Dartmouth running community. Several weeks passed, and then Rachel reached out to me one night asking if we could meet for coffee the next day in New York City if I was in town. I immediately responded with the white lie that yes, I was around, and I'd love to meet. In reality I was at a race in Boston— but as soon as I finished competing, I skipped my flight back to Oregon and hitched a ride with a runner I met that night at the race to get me to the city the next morning. We drove through the night together and got to NYC just in time. I stayed up all night and it was so worth it. I think if Rachel had known what I went through to make it to our meeting, she wouldn't have felt comfortable asking me to meet—but I didn't want any logistical obstacles in the way of actually getting to spend time with this woman I so admired. Rachel was my dream movie-mom.

Knowing I may never be in the same room as people has never stopped me from making them into mentors. I've learned how to look up to women I admire from afar, which takes the same kind of imagination my little-girl self used when I pretended someone else's mom was mine. For instance, even though I've never met Melissa Clark, I feel like I've drawn as much comfort from watching her *New York Times* food videos as I did from watching Kati's mom cook. When I watch Melissa's videos I pretend she is my mom telling me how to make a crumble— joking that it doesn't really matter if the strawberries are chopped perfectly because people don't like perfect! If you're feeling brave, add mint! She taught me that it is better to be brave, not perfect. With Melissa, I always try to listen to what she's actually saying beneath the recipe itself. What she means when she says she is going to save the crisp edges of the casserole for herself is that she values herself enough to give herself the best part of her creation. She is kind to herself first.

Britney Spears is another example: she taught me to unapologetically commit to my goals after I read in a magazine that as a child she used to take over the family bathroom to sing into her hairbrush because she knew she was destined to be a singer when she grew up. She took her dreams seriously and I latched on to that idea like a barnacle.

And there were others. I listened to the audio edition of Tina Fey's book *Bossypants* twice in one week because when I found out that she is Greek like me, I decided that she could be my mentor, too. When she talks about the way she looks, I thought, that's the way that *I* look, and that made me feel more capable of becoming someone like her.

When I was little other people believed that I lacked something because of my mother's death. I can never know for sure exactly what I missed out on. But what I *do* know is that her death forced me to seek out female mentorship on my own terms, and the mother-shaped hole in my heart has now been filled by wonderful women of my choosing. My greatest loss has become my greatest gift: I've learned that the whole world and all its inhabitants are there for me to observe, absorb, and imitate. I will never outgrow or be too proud for mentors.

Even though my mother's experiences are forever closed to me, the rest of the world is wide open. Like a buffet, I want all the shrimp, all the pasta, and all the chocolate fondue. I don't have the one person; I have every person. I can pick and choose bites of anything. My selections might not all make sense on the plate together, but I crafted this meal; it is mine, and I love it.

the cake pretends

to be a cake

before it is baked.

desiring the joining of

a world of butter and sugar

milk friends flour

it begs the heat please

without lumps or complaint

alter and whole

the thick into shape

recognizably cake.

by making itself

believe

it is saying

"i could be a cake."

PUBERTY POWER

My family and I stood together in the small waiting room just outside the Oval Office, nervously smiling like a group of kids waiting their turn at the top of a waterslide. My brother, Louis, stood at the front of our pack, ready to walk in first—he had spent the past few years working on President Obama's staff and this was his last day on the job. As such, he was invited to bring his family for a meet-and-greet with Obama himself. The Oval Office door cracked open and laughter spilled out into the waiting room. The family ahead of us walked out, and there he was: the president of the United States, standing just a few feet away.

One by one, we shook President Obama's hand. Louis introduced me as a professional runner. This was in 2015, before I was an Olympian. President Obama's attention turned to me. "You have a gift," he said. "You were born with a body that was meant to run long distances, more than the average human."

Right away I knew what I wanted to say in response . . . but dare I risk embarrassing my brother by disagreeing with President Obama, his former boss and the most powerful person in the country, a man we both admire and revere? I started by thanking the president, and then I couldn't help myself—I added that my performance in the sport was just a result of hard work, motivation, and support from my community. But the president disagreed.

"No, no," he said. "Your body is able to flush out lactic acid better than the average person—running is what you were born to do." Obama's energy and tone was so confident and convincing that he could have told me the moon is really made out of cheese and I would have agreed with him. I nodded and thanked him. Besides, our five-minute meeting time was up. I left the Oval Office feeling very honored, but I also couldn't stop thinking about what the president had said. The idea that I was meant to run, that I was born with a special ability, felt like it subtracted from my own willpower and motivation.

My brother later told me that President Obama was a serious basketball player as a teenager and competed on one of the best high-school teams in the country. He grew up training tirelessly, presumably with big basketball dreams, and it wasn't until later that he hung up his jersey and focused his attention elsewhere—though basketball was still near and dear to his heart. The thing was, as Obama grew up, he discovered that there were physical barriers that prevented him from advancing to compete at the highest level of basketball. No matter how hard he worked, he wasn't as tall or fast or coordinated as his competitors. That must have been deeply frustrating and heartbreaking to someone as driven and disciplined as President Obama. Could that explain his comments about my body's natural ability to run long distances?

* * *

In middle school and early high school, it's safe to say that natural ability was a huge factor in my athletic prowess. With a wiry body and unusually long limbs, I managed to become one of the top young runners in California. I finished fourth in the state my sophomore year. At the same time, I was also developing an interest in other things—student government, theater, competitive soccer, and a social life. But being a well-rounded teenager was not what my high school's athletic leadership wanted.

At the beginning of junior year, my track coach, along with the head of my high school's athletic department, gave me an ultimatum: I would need to quit soccer or I would be kicked off the track team. He felt it was right and best to force high-school athletes to specialize. The system itself was structured to benefit athletes who specialized and punish those with a diversity of commitments. Not all athletes, to be clear—only female athletes. There were multi-sport male athletes at our school who were celebrated, but for some reason the women's running coach (who was a man) felt that we needed to erase the other parts of our identities to succeed, as if a fifteen-year-old girl who had to miss a few practices represented a threat to the athletic department's authority. They wanted me to be a compliant good girl. I wasn't a bad girl, but I wanted to be treated respectfully. There was not a single woman in this whole conversation—the entire school leadership was men. My father and I made an official complaint to the school leadership but we were disregarded. My dad even consulted with a lawyer, but ultimately decided not to pursue the case because private Catholic schools have minimal accountability beyond their own internal decision-making. Had this happened today, I'm sure it could have become a viral moment that would have stoked outrage. This was the most potent encounter with sexism I've ever had in my life—being unabashedly told that I was being held to a different standard than the boys within the high-school athletic system.

Since I didn't want to quit soccer, I was not allowed to be on the cross-country or track teams and I didn't run that year. Then, in senior year, I tried to re-join the cross-country team. The coach once again made it clear that he would not permit anyone to miss or reschedule anything, especially if the conflict was with any other extracurricular activities. This came to a head for me during Spirit Week, which is a very big deal at Bishop O'Dowd High School. It is the biggest week of the year, full of themed days and bonding activities. During Spirit Week each grade was responsible for decorating a section of hallway in a particular theme. And when I say "decorate," I mean it was tradition to *cover* your entire section with a full 3-D set. We were the "Super Nintendo Seniors." We had worked for weeks on the hallway decorations and, as the class vice president, I was personally responsible for ensuring that the decorations went up in time. I asked my coach to let me miss practice for a day so that I could be there during the final pre–Spirit Week decorating push, but he said no, I had to be at practice, and if I wasn't there then I'd be kicked off the team. I missed practice and that was that—the end of my high-school running career.

I wish the coach would have seen that as a high schooler, I did not feel ready to specialize in anything, especially a sport that I was good at but had not yet fallen in love with. I was slowly learning to enjoy running, but it was not for the reasons he was trying to force on me. I was a late bloomer; I always have been. And I was gradually growing into the sport just as I was gradually growing into myself. The things I liked about running were the moments when sport felt *fun*. Like when my pals on the team and I would secretly divert from our forty-five-minute run and jump in the reservoir instead. We'd come back dripping wet and tell the coach "It was just so hot out there, we sweated so much!" Or the nights when we'd buy giant blocks of ice from the 7-Eleven and sneak into the golf course next to the park where we trained. Someone would sit on the block long enough that a little seat was melted into it and we'd take turns sliding down the grassy hills. For Bay Area kids, this was the closest we ever got to sledding in our hometown. Don't get me wrong, we trained hard enough. We were one of the best teams in the state. But we were also teenagers. The minute the coach set unreasonable boundaries for us, it stopped being fun and started feeling too serious. All the joy was gone.

The focus of high-school sports should be on human development, not high achievement. Competition results are a by-product, not the end goal. I'm glad my father never pushed me to specialize in running at a young age—he and I both knew I was good, but my dad's top priority was seeing me thrive as a person. He'd rather me be a happy normal kid than a stressed-out running star. I wanted to experience things. I was in the school play, I partied, I drank, I experimented. Nothing too extreme, but probably not the type of behavior most parents would associate with a future Olympian. If you look at a snapshot of me in any one moment of my high-school life, you probably wouldn't guess where I would end up.

The ironic twist is that my forced retirement from high-school running became a major advantage in my later growth as an NCAA and then professional athlete. I inadvertently stopped training just long enough for my body to go through puberty without the strain of overtraining, which is exactly the challenge that most girls in distance running face at that age.

The vast majority of athletic programs, even at the collegiate level, lack the most fundamental information about how to properly guide female athletes through puberty and young adulthood. Programs confuse *health* with *fitness*. Fitness is not an indicator of durability and sustainability; it is only an indicator of athletic ability at the present moment. Health, on the other hand, is a more holistic measure of the body's functionality over time. Fitness does not take into account that you need to continue training tomorrow and next week. It is better to be a hundred percent healthy and eighty percent fit than a hundred percent fit and eighty percent healthy.

But that's not the way most programs see things. Fitness is rewarded while health is taken for granted. I don't think this approach always comes from a bad place, it just comes from ignorance—and the unfortunate result is that when female athletes hit puberty, they'll often take shortcuts to fitness at the expense of their long-term health. When a girl's body transitions from adolescence into adulthood, the physical changes that occur can seem—at first—to be counterproductive to fitness, mainly weight gain as her frame expands and her body fills out. I once consoled a college teammate after the coach called her into his office and made her hold a five-pound weight in each hand and pump her arms as if she was running, and then had her put the weights down and pump her arms again—a demonstration of how much easier it is to run after losing ten pounds.

So in an effort to please their coaches and keep up with their male teammates, whose developmental trajectory is completely different, many female athletes overtrain and don't eat enough during this critical growth phase instead of allowing puberty to naturally take its course. (I know female athletes whose periods were delayed until their twenties.) One of the upperclassmen on my high-school track team—we'll call her Blythe—is a classic example of overtraining and underfueling. By the time she was a senior, Blythe was hospitalized for an eating disorder. But for months and even years, she got away with it. The thing about eating disorders in distance running is that, for a window of time, they appear to be effective—until they aren't. While other girls were filling out and running slower times, Blythe was thin and muscular and as fast as ever . . . until she broke.

When I joined the team as a freshman, Blythe saw me as a threat to her reign as one of the fastest girls in school and she actually became a bully. During a practice the day after I'd beaten her in a race, she made all the boys run the opposite direction as me on the track. I felt bewildered and lame. Another time, she convinced me to run intentionally slower during a race, and yet another time, she manipulated me into forfeiting a state championship race that she herself did not qualify for. I was younger, confused, and impressionable. She was not a good role model. I now understand that she must have been suffering tremendously at the time, but back then it was hard for me to have a teammate who wasn't eating and who based her entire sense of worth on how fast she was in any given season.

The result of this systemic prioritization of fitness over health for young female athletes is that many girls will become frail and injury-prone by the time they're in college—as a result of her eating disorder, Blythe had injuries for almost her entire collegiate career. I know this because we went to rival colleges and I saw her show up to race after race in a medical boot. The athletic system failed Blythe and then she failed me. That's the thing about faulty systems; they will ruin individuals who then, in turn, pass the harm along to the next batch of people.

It breaks my heart to think of all the young women who quit the sport because the system made them feel as if they "weren't built for distance running." To me, that is the biggest tragedy, when somebody gives up on a dream because of being mishandled or otherwise rushed due to a system that does not work. When the same bad things happen to a group of people time and time again, it is important to look closer at the failed system that is responsible. We are failing ourselves if we don't.

* * *

After I stopped running my junior year, my coaches assumed that I'd be lost to the vortex of puberty that claims so many female runners. But what none of them knew is that rather than being a death sentence, puberty is a superpower. The body that I grew during my junior and senior years of high school was capable, durable, and powerful because I wasn't fighting against my body's natural inclinations. I grew C-cup boobs. I rode the puberty wave and then, when the time was right, I gradually increased my training. My mature body was far more durable and powerful and capable than the twisted Peter Pan prepubescent body that most female athletes feel pressured to maintain. It is a problem to assume that if we allow a girl to go through normal body maturity, she will never again be as capable as she was prepuberty. It's straight-up wrong, because in reality, most female distance runners peak in their late twenties and early thirties. Our bodies take time to develop. Why can't *develop* be a word we embrace?

This systemic misunderstanding of the female distance-running trajectory extends into the professional world, too. In one of my first meetings with a potential sponsor, when I was fresh out of college, the male CEO behind a female-branded athletic apparel company offered me a generous contract and told me that if, in a few months, he felt that it was smart for me to retire, he would be the first to tell me and I could keep my contract by making ads for the company instead of competing. He framed it as if he was doing me a favor, this man in his sixties telling a twenty-one-year-old woman that he would decide when she was past her prime. He fundamentally misunderstood that I was actually at the beginning of my athletic potential, not the end. He was in no position to deem my body incapable at such a young age. His diagnosis of my performance limits stemmed from an understanding of the sport based on the male athletic trajectory, which has nothing to do with the natural progression of the female athlete's body. Maybe he was basing his information on his experience of watching so many female athletes fall apart in their early twenties thanks to the system that overtrained them through puberty, but that wasn't the case for me.

I steadied my voice to explain to him that I wanted to be an Olympian. That I did not want to quit in the next few months, as he thought might be the case. I had just committed to my Olympic dream and the last thing I needed was this man telling me when my time was up. We did not end up working together. It turns out I dodged a major bullet: This same CEO later grabbed my waist and grinded up on me from behind without asking when he was drunk at an industry party during the National Club Cross Country Championships. He creepily said that he was "sorry things didn't work out between us." It made me really uncomfortable to be touched and spoken to in this way and I felt sorry for all the athletes who felt inclined to "dance" with him that night because he was their boss. I left the event immediately, uncomfortable to even be in the same space as him—later, one of his top athletes reached out to my coach to apologize on his behalf.

From my draconian high-school coach to this CEO, I learned firsthand that the distance running world is not structured to embrace female athletes. But it doesn't have to be this way. Starting as early as middle and high school, we can educate coaches and athletes on the proper approach that young women can take to embrace their bodies and stay healthy and ultimately grow into more capable adults. I had two incredible female coaches in my career, Maribel Souther at Dartmouth and Maurica Powell at the University of Oregon, both of whom showed by example what a thriving female athlete could be. I hope that as more women take leadership roles in the athletic world, it can one day become common knowledge that female bodies operate on different performance timelines than their male teammates and require a different type of support.

* * *

When I started college, it was expected that I would join the cross-country team. Dartmouth's recruiters had reached out to me on the basis of my performance my sophomore year of high school, and the coach was interested in my potential. I also saw a future for myself in running and I liked the idea of committing to a sport where I could do some damage. I was curious. And unlike the coaches who wanted me to specialize in high school, in college I found a coach and team who inspired me instead of pressured me. I felt ready and even happy to embrace running.

But when I reported to my first practice, it became abundantly clear that I would no longer breeze to the top of the ranks as I had in middle school and early high school. I couldn't rely on my talent alone. After two years away from competitive running, my body had changed. It was humiliating to have to walk after only a few miles on easy training runs while my teammates literally ran circles on the trails around me. I finished dead last in my first cross-country race. I was not only the last on my team; I had one of the slowest times in the whole league. After each of my bad races, some of my older teammates took me out to a cave-themed bar that we knew would serve underage students. Nobody else drinking in that bar at noon (cross-country races were morning events) expected me to do anything great, so it was easy to not expect anything of myself, either.

Running wasn't the only part of college life I struggled with: My adjustment to Dartmouth's academics felt like falling into an ice-cold lake—it was a shock and I could barely keep my head above water. Unlike the kids who either came from high-end prep schools *or* were just straight-up geniuses, which it seemed like most of my new classmates at Dartmouth were, I soon realized that my high-school academic experience left me drastically underprepared for the rigors of an Ivy League education. One of my professors called me in for a special meeting after I failed yet another multiple-choice midterm and asked if I might have a learning disability. Anytime I failed a test, I had a sad little tradition where I'd take myself out to Ramunto's, a pizza spot in Hanover, and treat myself to several garlic-knot pizza slices, where the crust is actually made of garlic knots. I ate at Ramunto's more often than I'd like to admit.

I knew that, like my fitness, my grades wouldn't magically improve on their own. It was going to take hard work. I visited my professors outside of class nearly every day to review the questions I got wrong on a test or how I could improve an essay. And slowly, over time, I learned how to be an Ivy League student. I learned how to focus during long lectures and how to write an analytical essay. I feel grateful that I had the intellectual capacity to teach myself these things, but I certainly would have failed out of Dartmouth without an incredible amount of hard work. The same principle held true with my running: My athletic talent was there, but it needed to be molded by hard work.

Those first few semesters in college were a long trudge toward getting my fitness back. In time, six-mile runs became ten-mile runs, and six hours of sleep became nine. I stopped failing tests, so garlic-knot pizzas phased out of my regular routine. I stopped going to bars to drown my sorrows after tough races, both because I now had younger teammates looking up to my example and because I learned that one night of heavy drinking would set me back about two weeks' worth of training. Since I valued my time and was becoming more serious about my running, I became much pickier about when I chose to drink. My improv group, The Dog Day Players, had late-night shows a few times a week at various frat and sorority houses, and I learned to hang out with non-running friends after the shows without drinking. Did you know if you just carry around a cup, even if it's only filled with water, nobody will ask why you aren't drinking? I came to really enjoy having a well-rounded college experience on my own terms.

I also learned more about nutrition. In my dad's house, food was just food. He never used words like *healthy* or *unhealthy*, just like he never used words like *pretty* or *ugly*, which I appreciate deeply. I didn't have harmful complexes about food, for which I am very grateful, but I also didn't have basic knowledge of how to fuel properly.

Food can be a sensitive subject for female distance runners, harkening back to the pressure that most girls face to stay thin even as their bodies are desperately trying to develop and mature. At Dartmouth, some girls on my team made a practice of limiting their portions by only eating from the palm-sized side-dish bowls in our cafeteria, never actual plates. When I became captain, I instituted a rule that you had to eat proper portions off a real plate. At UO, there was a teammate who ate all her meals with chopsticks, one grain of brown rice at a time. Every team at every school has cases like this (my friend at Brown reported that her coach had a "no booze, no boys, no bagels" policy), and I don't know exactly what the right answer is for athletes who struggle with weight. It's true that for each person, there *is* an optimal "race weight range"—but I believe that for female runners especially, coaches and athletes should take more factors than just weight into account. Longevity and durability should be part of the conversation as well. And it *should* be a conversation; we should not be silent about food.

In the meantime, while I was not fit enough to contribute to the team in a competitive sense, I contributed in other ways.

When the traveling squad went to New York City for the Ivy League Cross Country Championships, I found my own transportation to the race and went in costume to cheer them on. My costume was a full snakeskin bodysuit and I cheered at the top of a big hill alongside a boy from Brown dressed as the Burger King, mask and all. In this way, even when I was not fit enough to score a team point, I could still find ways to matter by staying engaged, leaning in, and contributing any way I knew how. It built my self-worth and gave me a purpose every day while my body caught up. It takes integrity, determination, humility, and, most of all, a sense of humor to be the team mascot when just a few years earlier I would have easily beaten any of these girls. I kept showing up and I'm proud of how I handled myself during those few years. Yes, years. It wasn't until the winter of my junior year that I contributed my first team point.

In my senior year, I competed in an NCAA Track and Field Championship for the first time. By then, the preternaturally talented prepubescent Alexi who placed high in state championship meets as a tween was long gone. The new Alexi was made from endless work, discipline, patience, and pain (and lots of sleep). Stepping up to the start line for the first leg of the distance medley relay at the 2012 NCAA Indoor Championships felt like something I had fought for and earned. I even got matching tattoos with my relay teammates because we were so proud. We had set a lofty goal, worked hard, and made it happen.

When I became a professional runner, my first coach paired me with Sally Kipyego, an Olympic silver medalist, as a training partner. For that entire season, I would either shit my pants, throw up, or otherwise have to stop at some point during every single workout. We had two workouts per week and I never finished one all the way through, and that was by design. I was in a program where I was meant to keep up with my training partner until my body gave out, and then the workout was done for me. I ran twice a day almost every day, more than a hundred miles total a week, plus we lifted weights and had drill sessions at least two to three times per week. It was an unprecedented level of athletic commitment and exertion.

I am grateful that I had the opportunity to safely and naturally grow a body durable enough to withstand that level of effort. I'm certain that if I had never gone through puberty and menstruated normally, my body would have broken down after just a few workouts in the professional world.

I'm also grateful that I had the natural talent somewhere inside me to develop into a world-class runner, as President Obama said. I appreciate that someone else might have worked just as hard as me without achieving the same results. But if talent gave me a powerful engine, then hard work is my fuel. An engine is useless without the fuel.

I don't know if being a good athlete comes down to being born gifted or working hard. We can't know; it is always some combination of the two. I would also contend that a third factor, *health,* is an equally important ingredient for athletic success. I hope that in the future, new generations of female runners will come of age in an environment that sets them up for long-term durability. Because no matter how powerful the engine and how potent the fuel, the whole thing is useless if it burns out too soon.

Braveys, the biggest takeaway is this: We can't control the engine we're given. But how we treat our engine is entirely up to us. It will take us to the moon if we let it.

chasing a dream is like building a sandcastle.

every grain of sand is important, even if you
can't see them all.

MY PAL, PAIN

To qualify for the Olympics, it is important to become a master of pain. At the 2016 Olympics in Rio de Janeiro, I ran the 10,000 meters—twenty-five laps, the longest race on the track. It's a grueling combination of endurance running and speed. It's a test of pain tolerance and mental toughness as much as of athletic ability.

Throughout nearly the past decade of serious running, I've come to trust that I can exert myself to my absolute physical limit, and I will (most likely) not die. Deep down, I knew the difference between athletic pain, which is good pain, and other kinds of pain, bad pain. Whatever pain I felt while I was wearing running shoes could never be as bad as the things I had seen my mom do. Bad pain was scary; good pain just hurt.

But just because I have a high tolerance for pain doesn't mean I enjoy it. In middle and high school, I dreaded every single race. Not because I was anxious about finishing well but because I was terrified of the pain that came with it. I had a very specific daydream that I would entertain before every race: An alien spaceship would land in the middle of the track right before the starting gun and I would get to go home. Nobody could ever make us run after such a dramatic extraterrestrial disruption. But no matter how much I fantasized, the Martians never came and the starting gun always fired—followed by the inevitable onset of pain.

I have never been able to fully recall the exact sensations of pain during those races, but I do remember certain details, gestures of pain. Salt-sweat residue chafing between my legs, my vision blurring with sunscreen, a pool of sweat gathering between my thick eyebrows, which furrowed so deeply they fused with my poorly mascaraed eyelashes. My entire body was an ant farm swarming with pain, transparent and open, my suffering on display for all to see.

Despite days of anxiously anticipating races, the pain still shocked me every time it arrived. I would think back wistfully to all the times when I *wasn't* in pain and scold myself for not being grateful enough for every leisurely second watching cartoons, eating fried calamari, or doing *anything* besides running.

After every single race ended, even when I won, my joy at finishing was tainted by the trauma of the pain I had just experienced. I would stomp directly from the finish line over to my dad, who I remember as having a camera for a nose, and report to him that seriously, this race could have killed me, and I simply could *not* go through this again. My dad would say the same thing every time: "It's okay, Lex."

When I went to college and started training to compete at the Division 1 level, intense pain became part of my daily routine. Every morning I woke up dreading the inevitable pain to come and by the time practice started, I felt mentally drained. It became clear that if I wanted to survive as a college runner, I needed to develop a technique to manage my fears about pain. I could no longer afford to spend the days leading up to workouts and races steeped in anxiety. Negative thinking drains energy, and I needed all the energy I had to keep up with my new team-mates. Pain and I had to come to a new understanding.

I thought back to middle school when I got into a fight with this girl I really didn't get along with. When our teacher finally intervened, she quarantined us in a room called "the pod" for an hour to figure things out, just us two eleven-year-olds. My ad-versary and I spent a good forty-five minutes in silence, glaring at each other from under our unibrows. But in the end we agreed that while we didn't want or need to be friends, we could be civil for both our sakes. I resolved to be similarly civil with pain. Before my races and big workouts, I worked on con-sciously shifting my mental energy from dreading upcoming pain to simply recognizing that the pain would always show up no matter what, and even though I utterly despised it, I should try to greet it politely like a guest at a dinner party and be fully prepared to open the door when it does. Sometimes pain arrives slowly, like butter melting on toast. Or it can be quick, like but-ter hitting a very hot pan. Whichever variety of pain I'm get-ting, I know it is coming and I am prepared to handle it gracefully.

The next step was to teach myself to manage the pain once it arrived. Visualization became my most powerful tool: I learned to anticipate which parts of a race would be the most grueling, either by studying the course beforehand or talking to people who had run the race before. In the days leading up to the race, while jogging, cutting my nails, or scrambling eggs, I'd visualize an Alexi-inside-my-head approaching a specific painful moment along the course and pushing through the rough patch with composure, strength, and even beauty. When I actually faced the challenge in the race, I knew the pain was coming—and, most crucially, I had already made the decision to persevere.

I also discovered using physical triggers, *playable actions*, as a tool to help my mind overcome the anxiety associated with the onset of pain. For example: "When the pain hits after the third mile, remember to shake your arms out and drop your shoulders." Or even something as simple as: "When it hurts, force yourself to smile." By converting a mental struggle into an actionable objective, internal battles felt less elusive and more grounded. It's much easier to tell myself to move my arms than it is to tell myself to "feel better."

After I finished school, I started running professionally with my eye on competing in the Olympics. Thrust into this new world of elite runners, I had a surprising realization: My competitors were all experiencing pain, too. I idolized pro runners when I was growing up and I assumed that these mythical creatures must have figured *something* out about pain that I hadn't. There's no way that these professionals hurt as much as I did. But now that I was up close to this new tier of athlete, I saw that I wasn't the only one struggling. As it turns out, running hurts for everyone.

At the top level, everyone has their own method for managing pain. Some runners wear their pain openly while others hide it very well. But in the same way that it's usually unhelpful to compare my life to how other people's lives look on their Instagram feeds, I had to stop comparing myself to how other people in my races looked. Looks can be deceiving, and more often than not, we try to show only the most glamorous parts of ourselves.

I remember in one of my first competitions as a post-collegian, I found myself running side by side with an accomplished Olympian who maintained a calm face and strong posture despite our grueling pace. I felt intimidated—was this woman not in pain? But then halfway through the race, she suddenly fell behind the pace and completely dropped back, seemingly out of the blue. I'd been so sure that her steady breathing meant that I was alone in my suffering, when in truth she must have been feeling even more pain than I was. Without a doubt, I learned that day that pain is the one thing my competitors and I definitely have in common.

My deeper understanding of physical pain has helped me cope with emotional pain, too. First of all, I know that pain shows up differently for each person and I can never tell just how much somebody else might be hurting. I also understand that whenever I feel bad, I'm probably not alone. I may not always know when emotional pain is coming, and I do get sad sometimes—I get bouts of sadness that come out of nowhere and feel like a sorbet scoop to the heart. Sometimes it's related to a memory of my mom, and sometimes it doesn't have any reason for being at all, but I am equipped to greet the sadness when it arrives.

When I was unexpectedly quarantined in Greece for five months during the COVID-19 pandemic (I initially planned to spend only the month of February 2020 there for pre-Olympic training), I had nothing to do but train very hard since my support network there was just my Greek coach. I was already in an emotionally vulnerable place, on account of just learning that the Olympics had been postponed by a year and that I'd be away from my family for an unknown amount of time, when during

one very challenging and windy workout, my Greek coach
started yelling at me like I'd never been yelled at before. He was
screaming at the top of his lungs to be heard over the wind. This
wasn't anything new, shouting was just his style, but suddenly I
felt a tidal wave of unexpected sadness. His yelling, which felt
completely unmerited and disproportionate to the situation at
hand, woke something up inside of me related to the little-kid
memories of my mom screaming at the top of her lungs in the
kitchen. Back then I had to hold everything inside, but now I
allowed myself to burst into tears as I continued the workout.
Crying was my *playable action*.

I think this is called grief, feeling and even embracing your
painful feelings. Pain needs to see itself in the mirror and *be felt*
before it can go away. When I feel sad and I hold it in, I feel
completely alone. But when I let it out, I let go of all pretenses.
I'm just a human, which is comforting because it means that I'm
not alone. It's good to grieve. After my workout in Greece, I had
a talk with my coach and explained that I'm already hard
enough on myself, and as an athlete I respond best to calm confidence rather than passionate yelling. Coach was wonderfully
understanding.

All pain takes its time. Some hurt fades quickly, but other
times it lingers like the glop of powder stuck at the bottom of a
mug of hot chocolate. No matter what kind of pain I am confronted with, I have a choice about how I interact with it and
how I let it affect me. But *all* pain, whether it's the physical kind
you feel during a race or the quieter kind you feel in normal life,
gets better with time. Just remember: All marshmallows, when
squeezed, can reinflate eventually.

grit is what's left over when nothing's left

COACH IAN

I first met Coach Ian shortly after he retired from a successful Olympic running career, which in itself made him a good coach; he had accomplished what he needed to accomplish in his own career, so his coaching career was just about being there for his athletes. Even though he was young for a coach, he had no ego to satisfy. He also knew what it took to achieve the loftiest goal of all, making an Olympic team.

Just as much as I believed in Ian, he believed in me. When I was with him, whether alone or in a packed stadium before a race, I felt like I had everything I needed to succeed. That mutual belief fueled our relationship.

There is a way that a coach and athlete love each other, which is a kind of love that's not like any other. It revolves around a shared goal where each person plays a very specific and important role. An athlete and a coach complete each other. An athlete has to learn how to get the most out of herself and also how to draw support and wisdom from the reservoir that is her coach. And the coach must learn how to best support, teach, and protect the athlete, and also when to push the athlete to the edge of her ability.

I trusted Coach Ian to know my potential and my limits. He knew when to hold me accountable and when to push me harder, and he also knew when to listen to my complaints and evaluate if something was truly wrong. There were days that he made me take my watch off and continue the workout without obsessing over pace, and there were days when he'd look me in the eye and tell me this was a workout where I needed to suck it up and hit the pace no matter how much it hurt because he knew I could. And then there were days when he saw that I just needed to step off the track and go home. There was as much laughter as tears, as much grace as grit. Ian knew when to push, when to pull, and when to leave me alone. I have always known that I have a dangerously high tolerance for pain. But the same tolerance that helps me win might also allow me to hurt myself. Ian made me feel like I was totally safe pushing myself, like a kite allowed to fly higher and higher but always safely held by trustworthy hands at the other end of its string. It is a gift to not have to question yourself while working on your goals.

One day, after a rough workout, I was beating myself up because I couldn't hit the pace I should have. I felt frustrated and even a little bit afraid, since the Rio Olympics were just around the corner. I thought my slow workout meant that I was failing. But then Coach Ian gave me the best advice I've ever gotten: It's called the Rule of Thirds. When you're chasing a big goal, you're supposed to feel good a third of the time, okay a third of the time, and crappy a third of the time. If the ratio is off and you feel good all the time, then you're not pushing yourself enough. Likewise, if you feel bad all the time, then you might be fatigued and need to dial things back.

Learning the Rule of Thirds was life-changing for me, not

only as an athlete but also as a creative, as someone in a relationship, and as a person in general, because it made me believe in the days that didn't feel great. In fact, I relished them, knowing that even those days were an important part of the process. The hard days just meant that I was chasing a dream. It mattered that it was Coach Ian who told me about the Rule of Thirds—where advice comes from can be just as important as the advice itself, and any advice coming from an admired mentor carries tremendous significance.

In Rio, before my Olympic race, security measures prevented Coach Ian from being in the athletes' warm-up area, where he'd typically post up. So we set a meeting spot just off to the side of the athletes' entrance, which was enclosed by a chain-link and barbed-wire fence. I saw him appear through a crowd of fans pouring into the stadium. He was holding a to-go coffee cup, which is his signature prop. There was chaos all around us. Ian was not allowed inside the fence, so this was the closest we'd get before the biggest race of my life. He put his fingers through the fence and interlocked them with mine. The minute we touched I was overwhelmed with the emotion of all the things we'd experienced together, the years we spent nurturing this Olympic dream and building it brick by brick. The first thing Ian said to me was, "Did you find some good coffee?," which for me is a prerace ritual only he would know to ask about.

Then he told me *I could do it*. He said he would be one of the dots in the thousands of people in the crowd. Then he did something I'd never seen him do before: He cried a little. I cried, too. Then the guards told Coach Ian it was time to move away from the fence. He said goodbye and joined the people in the stadium who were all eagerly anticipating the start of the race. I stood at the fence alone for a moment until the reality set in that I was on my own. It was up to me to do this thing that Coach Ian and I had spent years preparing for together. But I also realized that I was ready. Before that moment, I honestly didn't know if I'd ever feel ready to race in the Olympics, but as I watched Ian walk away, I knew I was.

A good coach does not worry about letting you grow up right in front of them. Because a good coach knows you will. That's what a coach does: They get you ready and then they let you go.

all i want

is to give it

all i got

THE OLYMPICS

The 2016 Olympics, and especially the Olympic Village, felt like a giant summer camp that brought the world's most athletic bodies and minds together in one place. And, like the first day of camp, I arrived in Rio feeling nervous. But instead of worrying about whether I'd packed the right kind of sandals, here it felt like my entire life's work was at stake. I wanted my race to go well, but in a more zoomed-out sense, I wanted very badly for my entire *Olympic experience* to go well. I knew from my coaches and mentors that the Olympics can be everything you imagined or they can fall short of your expectations. It's like meeting a celebrity that you've looked up to for your entire life. If you've always pictured them as this perfect dreamlike being, there's no way they can ever live up to your imaginary ideals. Disappointment is inevitable unless you meet them as they are.

When I arrived in the Olympic Village the first thing I noticed were the rows of tall, balconied apartment buildings. Every building (except the Team USA building, which opts to be low-key) was covered in flags from the country of the athletes living there—China, Qatar, Czech Republic. The Australian building even had a life-size kangaroo statue outside. Because of my Greek heritage, I was competing for Greece, and my team shared a building with Croatia, Algeria, and Ethiopia, among others. Upon entering our building the first thing I noticed was a clique of Croatian and Algerian coaches smoking cigarettes and jovially watching the Games on television from beanbag chairs while house music thumped loudly from a portable speaker. I accepted this reality with what I can only describe as a "new-summer-camp smile" plastered to my face—when you're overwhelmed, excited, and scared all at once. It's a disarming moment when you realize that you are not fully in control; you're plopped into a new environment that you cannot change.

For elite athletes, especially endurance athletes, control is extremely important. Our sleeping environment, meals, and even how we spend our downtime are all carefully calibrated and controlled. Now that I was in the Olympic Village, I had to smile politely and accept the fact that unless I wanted to confront an entire horde of strange coaches from Eastern Europe, there *would* be house music loudly playing in the lobby. It felt like a crossroads moment: Either I could try to hold tight to my idea of how things *should* be, or I could let go and embrace this new reality. That is the choice all Olympians must make: to try to sterilize the experience and treat it like any other competition, or to embrace it as something totally special and different. I knew that I could either let the Olympic chaos crush me or I could make it fuel me. So I decided to wear my new-summer-camp smile like a Bravey badge, and I went upstairs to find my room.

I had four suite mates, all of whom were on totally different eating and sleeping schedules. I was the only one who brought the proper outlet adapter and thus this tiny object was in high demand by suite mates wanting to charge their phones or straighten their hair. I didn't grow up with sisters and suddenly I had four. It was fun but overwhelming. I retreated to my room when it felt like too much, wrapping myself in my special Olympic-themed comforter. The comforters at every Olympics are designed with unique colors and graphics reflective of that particular Games' aesthetic. At the end of the Games, every athlete takes their comforter home—mine took up half a suitcase and I will treasure it forever.

Like a summer camp, the Olympic Village had a uniform. Athletes wore their full national team uniforms at all times—this was a requirement enforced by every national team's leadership. Each uniform had multiple components—sweats, warm-ups, T-shirts, shoes, the works—and each country's uniform had its own distinct look. The Italian uniforms were designed by Armani. France, Lacoste. Sweden, H&M. The Slovakians' sweats had colorful squiggly circles and squares printed on them that looked like they could have been designed by Lisa Frank. The Greek uniform was mostly Mediterranean blue, and I even got a Greek fanny pack. My favorite item was my rain jacket, blue with tiny white Greek keys printed all over it. My uniform was gigantic on me—the smallest item I had was a T-shirt that fell below my knees. But despite the size mismatch, when I wore my uniform, I felt like I belonged in this village of athletes.

So much of my life has been spent trying to belong—and that's often okay, because it means I'm stretching my boundaries. But this can also be very uncomfortable. During my junior year of high school, one of the girls from the popular clique—they even had a name, Pussy Power, or P Squared for short—

invited me to join their Halloween pregame party. I had my main group of best friends, and we were all smart and well-liked and partied enough, but the P Squared girls were a notch hotter and wilder than we were. I felt really happy to be invited to their party, but when I showed up, I realized they were all already drunk and also were wearing costumes. The party was the weekend before Halloween and I hadn't gotten the memo that costumes were mandatory. I felt embarrassed and a little out of place.

The girl who was hosting the party—let's call her Amelia—swooped in and held my hand in a way that made me feel included as she led me to her closet and selected a pair of boy-short underwear that was lined with rows of pink lace. Then she told me to take my shirt off so that I was only in a bra. She told me to put some of her high heels on, so I did. Finally, she held up a giant chain-link collar, the kind designed for big dogs, and slung it around my neck. It felt like a coronation. "There! You're a dog!" I was a very scantily clad dog. But this was all fine; this felt like inclusion. I was relieved to be rescued into inclusion in this way. Even though Pussy Power then asked me to take all of their group photos but didn't ask me to be in them, I felt lucky to be there.

Then we all went to a warehouse party in Berkeley and I felt great in my outfit. One of the Pussy Power girls notified me that a kissing contest had begun, and whichever one of us kissed the most people won. I was glad I had my costume. Whenever anyone asked what I was, I whipped around my giant chain and told them, "Duh, a dog." To which everyone nodded in admiring acceptance. So simple! The costume! So good! It was even fun to dance in, because you can toss the chain over someone else's shoulder and you are instantly linked. Amelia was a genius.

And then Amelia blacked in. I hadn't even realized she was blackout drunk until that moment. In the middle of the party, in front of everyone, she shrieked at me as only a drunk girl can: "That's Fufu's collar! Why are you wearing my DEAD DOG'S COLLAR?" I paused, caught red-handed in a crime I didn't know I had committed. Slowly, I told Amelia that she had given it to me. Remember? But she just pulled the chain off my neck and stormed away in tears. I guess she didn't remember putting it on me. I stood there in front of a now-silent crowd, everyone's eyes on me, wearing only underwear and heels and no dog collar, meaning, no costume. I wasn't mad. It was worse: I was humiliated. Needless to say, I did not win the kissing contest.

I look back on that memory now with infinite fondness for my then-self, but at the time I felt awful. I felt like I did not belong. Wearing my Greek national uniform at the Olympic Village felt like the exact opposite of being stripped of my costume at the Halloween party. It felt like I had arrived.

* * *

I never felt any negative external pressure to perform well in my race, but I desperately wanted it to go well. Not just for my own sake but also because I was the first female distance runner for Greece *ever* to make it to the Olympics in the 10,000 meters—nobody had run the qualifying time before. The Greeks have particularly strong national pride when it comes to the Olympics—after all, Greece is where it all began—and it is always the first country to enter the Olympic Stadium during the opening ceremony in the Parade of Nations.

As a dual citizen of the United States and Greece, I could have stated my athletic allegiance to either country, but competing for Greece gave me the opportunity to make a larger impact with my performance. I will always remember when I went to my first training camp in rural Greece. A group of young girls who were there to watch the boys play soccer instead fixated on me running around the perimeter of the field. They asked why I looked strong "like a boy" and could hardly believe it when I told them that I was an athlete—they had never been exposed to female athletes who looked like me before. A good result in my race, now just a few days away, would make big waves in Greece and mean so much to so many people. It might even spark a fledgling Olympic dream for a young girl who would never have considered sports otherwise, and that meant the most to me.

To pass the time, I spent an inordinate number of hours in the athlete village dining hall, a colossal white structure two football fields long that resembled a holiday cake roll. There were giant food stations that boasted tubs of quail eggs, passion fruit, and countless prepared foods and condiments from cuisines around the world. I learned the hard way that the giant bucket of yellowish stuff next to the cold cuts was not honey mustard, it was dulce de leche. I've never gotten over the novelty of always having a hot meal ready for me—and the dining hall was full of novelties.

The dining hall did not feel like the real world. To me, and I think to the other athletes, too, it was a safe haven away from everything. Just outside was the whirlwind of the Olympic

Games, with high stakes and scary potential and the eyes of the world on us, but in here was our womb, our space to eat and chill. Even the sound of the dining hall was calming, with the low hum of hundreds of quiet conversations bouncing around the walls. The walls were thick plastic—the structure was temporary, so it was more like a gigantic tent than anything else—and the ambient sound wasn't harsh and echo-y like you might imagine a huge room to be, it was soft and enveloping.

From the outside, the way most people normally see them on TV, Olympic athletes appear as though they're at the pinnacle of their existence, as if they're fully formed entities that are entirely self-actualized. For the lucky few, that characterization is accurate. But the truth is, most Olympians feel just as confused and uncertain about themselves and their future as the rest of us. The Olympics are more of a process than an event. Nowhere is that more evident than in the dining hall.

The dining hall was open twenty-four hours a day and it was the best place to people-watch. All of our sports and countries were different, but everybody has to eat. Whenever I was feeling nervous or lonely, the dining hall was where I'd go. I think it is nice to be around other heartbeats even if they don't speak your language and even if they don't notice you're there, sitting alone, two seats over, observing how differently they use their fork and knife. I craved the backdrop of people more than I craved actual interaction with them.

My favorite game to play in the dining hall to distract myself from my own nerves was to guess an athlete's sport by looking at them. There were so many different shapes and sizes of people, and I tried to guess their sport by the look of their body or by the kind of crew they were rolling with. A giant posse meant it might be a team sport—if all the same gender, then even more likely—which narrowed things down. But my guessing game didn't stop at what sport someone might play. That was just the beginning of my speculative rabbit hole. I liked to imagine how people lived their life outside of the Olympic Village. I drew conclusions about people based on how they walked and carried themselves. Some athletes navigated the dining hall carefully, slowly, and with their heads down. That meant they might be new or nervous, which made me feel better; even if I was nervous, at least I was not alone.

But the dining hall wasn't only filled with the nervous head-down, hood-up types. There were also the confident, social-looking athletes—the boisterous, gregarious types, often found in packs with their team. It's easier to feel confident when you have your team with you—sometimes, teams of athletes would burst into national chants or cheers, especially after a big competition, and everyone nearby would smile and watch, like when the waiters all gather around someone's table in a restaurant to sing "Happy Birthday."

But the athletes who really caught my eye were the ones who projected confidence even when they were alone. If someone was basically gliding about the dining hall, summoning their burger and their noodles onto the plate like a god, then I guessed they had been to the Olympics before and were coming from a place of experience and knowledge. These people made me feel hopeful simply because I was occupying the same rarified space as them—I'd see how confident they looked and I'd tell myself that I had earned my spot here just like them, so maybe I should let myself feel confident like them, too. I am always fishing for ways to feel more confident and at home in places where I'm nervous. The truth is, playing this guessing game about other people's lives was a way to craft a narrative that helped me relate to each person I saw. It helped me convince myself that I fit in. The more I was able to see myself in my peers, the more I felt a part of the Olympics, and the more I felt capable of doing something great there.

* * *

Before my 10,000-meter race at the track stadium, there was pandemonium behind the scenes. Performing well was just as much about surviving the journey to the start line as it was about the race itself. Dozens of races needed to go off exactly at their scheduled times, without exception—after all, each race was the most important race in its athletes' lives. Amid the endless serpentine hallways through the track stadium's backstage it seemed impossible that my competitors and I would get to where we needed to be without losing our hip numbers, losing our way, and losing our lunch.

There's a saying that races are won and lost in the warm-up areas, and it's true. Before a race, it is easier to lose confidence than to gain it. I could tell that some of my competitors left their confidence on the warm-up field by the way they hung their heads, like the bobbleheads my dad obsessively collected from baseball games. I remember he would grab my hand and navigate me through the crowds and up the switchback ramps at the San Francisco Giants' stadium, half a step too swift for my nine-year-old legs. As I navigated the labyrinthine tunnels beneath the Olympic track stadium, my mind took me to the Giants' stadium back home. There's a funny thing about stadium hallways: They all smell the same.

My competitors and I finally arrived in the first of two call rooms where we were to be processed ahead of the race. In the first call room, we had our equipment checked—my competitors and I exchanged nervous looks while taking out our special track spikes, which are basically ballet slippers with nails underneath, and lacing them up anxiously. I saw different shoe-tying techniques all around me, and for a moment I questioned my own lacing methods, but I knew better than to change anything that specific on race day.

Through a crack in the door I could see into the main stadium hallway where spectators wandered between events, buying popcorn and commemorative T-shirts. The people with their ice creams and hot dogs were completely unaware that thirty-seven restless athletes were behind a thin wall just a few feet away. I closed my eyes to quiet my mind, but I was interrupted by a poke from a lady who handed me my official race bib and instructed me on how to fasten it to my uniform. She had the eyes of someone who had seen countless anxious athletes before me: no-nonsense, but also thoughtful and caring beneath her strict demeanor. She was going to instruct but not help, like a mother bird firmly but lovingly throwing her chick out of the nest.

After fifteen endless minutes in the first call room, a tall man in a sweat-drenched white cotton shirt told us it was time to move to the second call room. He had the enthusiasm of a parent who does not want to be a chaperone on a school field trip. As we all walked to the next room, my mind switched back and forth between feeling ready and feeling wholly unprepared for the task ahead.

In the second call room, I adjusted my shoes one last time. I have an irrational fear of losing a shoe mid-race, and I've come to accept that no amount of experience or mental fortitude will soothe it. So I just tie my shoes insanely tight before a race so there's no room for fear in my feet, and I leave it at that.

The tall sweaty man in the white cotton shirt yelled: "Everybody take your clothes off! Uniforms only! Everybody! Clothes! Off! Now! GIRLS!" Each of us took off our sweats until we were down to just race buns, spandex, and track spikes.

Then the man gathered us and told us it was time to test the special timing chips implanted in our race bibs. We were instructed to scurry across a little timing test mat one by one. If the mat beeped, it meant our timing chip was activated. This was all communicated by physical pantomime, since there were so many language barriers among the thirty-seven athletes, which meant this sweaty man had to demonstrate by bounding across the little mat himself.

One by one, like a group of trained circus lions, we leapt across the timing mat. What we weren't told was that we could not go back—the mat was a one-way ticket to the trackside corral, the final prerace holding area. A wave of panic rippled through my competitors in the corral, as nobody had thought to bring their water bottles across the mat to the other side. Nobody, that is, except for me.

Just moments ago I had been a relatively low-profile young athlete among my thirty-six competitors, but suddenly I became the *One with the Water*. If I'd wanted to I could have hoarded this water like a secret power that only I controlled. But then a voice next to me piped up: "Can I have a sip?" It was Almaz Ayana, the runner from Ethiopia who went on to break the world record during our 10,000-meter race.

I hesitated for a moment. It would have been entirely fair and within my rights to turn everyone else's lack of water into an advantage for myself. A younger me might have felt this was an opportunity to get private payback for the feeling of "lack" I had growing up. But then I considered all the incredible generosity that people have shown me throughout my life—and I grew up before my own eyes as I watched myself hand my water bottle to Almaz. This happens sometimes, where you notice yourself subtly but meaningfully surpassing your own expectations. And in that moment, you redefine who you are for yourself. I am now someone who shares. Growing up isn't always passive and gradual; sometimes it can be active and very sudden. Almaz smiled at me, took a healthy sip of my water, and then passed it on to the next girl. In this moment, I felt better for each drop of water shared than I would have for each drop of water hoarded. I couldn't help but think: All of these women want to kick your ass in this race, but all of them are basically good. It's not really us against each other, it's us against the whole world, all those popcorn and hot-dog people in the stands and the millions of others watching from their couches. We're all about to go do this wild dance together.

Then, quite suddenly, the corral door opened and we walked out onto the bright track. After a lifetime of preparing, the moment was finally here. I took a few sprints up and down the straightaway while television cameras hovered above me like curious hummingbirds. I looked into one of the cameras and waved, picturing my grandparents on the other side of the lens. It was the same feeling as being backstage in one of my elementary-school class plays right before the curtain comes up. Running is also a performance: We go onto a stage in a costume and we are the spectacle. We even wear makeup. On race day I always wear far more makeup than I ever do in real life, because this is a performance and it's supposed to feel special. But with running, the biggest performance isn't what the audience sees— it's what goes on inside your own mind. It's an inward performance: How much pain can I handle today? For me, putting on race-day makeup isn't about how the world sees me; it's about how I see myself. My race-day makeup symbolizes that this day is unique. It means that I am about to try something brave.

After a few moments the cameras pulled back and a hush settled over the stadium. I walked to the start line, took my position, and waited. A breath of silence, and then . . . POP! The starting gun fired and we took off running. All of us were trying to run faster than we ever had before. This was it, our Olympic race. Everything in our lives before had led to this point.

* * *

My coach had given me a specific pace to run for the majority of the race and I stuck to our plan. I understood I would begin in the far back of the pack but that it would pay off in the end. This was absolutely the case, as I slowly picked off one girl, and then another, and another. I felt confident, controlled, and joyful. When you are truly prepared for a race it can feel like you're almost watching yourself run while you run. I felt at home among my newfound sisters. We were all in this together.

Then the girl behind me kicked me in the heel and stepped

on the back of my shoe. Then she kicked my heel again. And AGAIN. When something like this happens once, it's an accident. Twice, okay. But three or four times and we have problems. That's when I remembered that this was not a kumbaya campfire, this was a race, and dammit, I'm competitive.

The 10k is a race of attrition, so generally it's not a matter of who runs away with it early but more about who is left at the end. I was now about halfway through the race, at which point the goal is to hang in there and not do anything crazy, just conserve energy for the climactic final lap. I kept telling myself to "stay."

But then there came the moment when the hurt set in. Every race hurts, no matter what. If anybody tells you otherwise they're either lying or they simply don't try hard enough. Normally when the hurt sets in I tuck my head down, grit my teeth, and force myself to smile. Then I thought about my family somewhere in the audience and all the ups and downs they had weathered during my journey to get here. I thought about how if the pain overcame me and I really did die right then and there, it was okay because there was nothing else I'd rather be doing.

As I ditched the heel-kicker and approached the final lap, running faster than I ever had, I realized that this wasn't really about me versus *her*—meaning any individual girl in my race— nor was this about me versus the world at large. It was about *me versus me,* just like in middle school, running as fast as I can and then some. It was about enjoying the results of my hard work and all the help I got from the people I love. My mental fitness and physical fitness were completely in sync, peaking simultaneously. It felt like the steep climb that began when I was a freshman at Dartmouth, with the countless days of pain and commitment, had culminated all in this one moment of perfect harmony. "Me versus me" doesn't do this feeling justice either— it's not a *versus*. It's me *within* me and me *outside* of me. I was running around the track while looking at a miniature diorama version of myself running around the track and this image repeated in my heart to infinity. It felt like my mind could tell my body to do anything and it would do it. Some people call this flow, but I call it bliss.

* * *

When you cross the finish line at the Olympics, there is no dad or boyfriend or coach to catch you. They are somewhere beyond the barricade of security fences. The people who catch you are the women you just raced, all of you wobbly and confused and happy and sad at the same time, overwhelmed that this thing you've held in your mind forever has finally happened.

My competitors and I gave each other the kind of support I can only imagine women in utopia might give each other when one of them has their period for the first time. (In reality, I got my first period in the woods while at cross-country practice. I was with my friend Amy, who demonstrated what a pad was by using a fallen leaf.) At the Olympic finish line I felt like I was with a new kind of family, one that was born instantly but was actually a culmination of all of our lives.

I stood on the track and waited for the last runner to finish. I saw my results go up on the giant jumbotron: I ran 31:36, shattering my personal best and setting a new Greek national record. I felt elated; I had done my absolute best. I felt like an Olympian. When you finish a race like this, it is emotional. You probably cry. I cried. I cried because it was the end of something and the beginning of something else.

* * *

After the race, when the dust settled and I was alone in my twin bed in my Olympic Village dorm later that night, I felt uneasy. I didn't want my Olympic experience to be over. Luckily, I still had two whole weeks left before the closing ceremony. That was two more weeks at the Olympics before I'd have to pack my bags and return to the real world.

I was aware that each second at the Games was precious. I wanted to soak up everything, like a sponge cake where the syrupy glaze saturates each morsel, crumb, and divot. I wanted the full experience. I had a vague inkling that maybe I'd try again for the next Olympics, but I had seen enough star athletes end their careers unexpectedly early to know and fully appreciate that this Olympic opportunity may only come once in my lifetime. I began to understand why it is important to take the opportunities we have in life when we get them, because only yesterday and today are for sure.

I started walking around while listening to music to see the Olympic Village through the soundtrack of my own personal movie, but I also sometimes left my headphones in my backpack when I felt open enough to take in the unexpected. I made a schedule for myself each day that included eating, napping, and training, but also visits to places I wanted to experience. I went to the medical tent for an ice bath every day, and each time I made the decision to share a tub with someone from a different sport and a different country. While inquiring about the free dental exams, I met a volunteer doctor from Brooklyn. He said he had called the International Olympic Committee every day for a year to get the chance to live and work in the village. He also told me that the Olympic Village doctor and dentist offices were packed at all hours of the day because this was the first doctor's appointment many athletes and coaches from less-developed parts of the world had had in four years (since the last Olympics). The Olympics mean different things to different people. For some, they are a lifeline of sorts. The doctor explained this to me and I guess I was curious and friendly enough that he thought this meant I was interested in something more—he later sent me a text and invited me to hang out at the Olympic Village swimming pool. I never replied. I know what kinds of partying happened at the pool. I filed this memory away and used it as the spark of inspiration for my next movie, *Olympic Dreams*, a romantic comedy that I filmed with Jeremy Teicher and Nick Kroll at the Winter Olympics two years later.

I will admit that the Olympic Village is very romantic. I often saw athletes wandering hand in hand at sunset along the shoestring of waterways that laced among the twenty-odd residential buildings. Condom dispensers adorned with the catchphrase "Celebrate with a Condom!" in three different languages were ubiquitous, and there was some kind of condom fairy whose job was to roam around with a knapsack full of condoms to keep the dispensers well-stocked.

Once it was dark, the parties began—often in the pool outside my building, and always well past my bedtime. Morning walks of shame were not uncommon, with an athlete wearing mismatched country uniform pieces scurrying across one of the walkways between the thousands of balconies and waving flags.

Soon the closing ceremony was just one day away. It felt exactly like the last day of summer camp: Everyone knows this is the last day to have fun before the buses come to whisk us back to the abyss of the real world. I couldn't help but feel nervous that I had somehow not soaked it all in enough.

During this last day, when I was wandering the village alone with my thoughts and frankly feeling a bit sorry for myself, I came across the beauty salon. I had heard that there was a free exclusive salon for Olympic athletes. But the beauty salon puzzled me: Why would anyone want to get a makeover at the Olympics? I always wear makeup to the starting line, but like most obsessive athletes, this is a ritual I perform on myself. Still, the salon beckoned to me—and in the spirit of experiencing all the Olympics have to offer, I decided to partake.

I ventured inside. A man at the front desk took one look at me and sprang out of his chair as if he could sense that I hadn't had my hair or makeup done in a salon in a very, *very* long time. He introduced himself as Kiko and told me that he would make me look like Lady Gaga. Before Kiko would handle my hair with his own hands, though, he asked me to comb it. He suspected that this was a battle best handled by me. I took the brush and began ripping through the many knots that dotted my head like holiday lights. I forced the brush from scalp to tip like a freight train bursting through piles of snow on the tracks. If a chunk of hair wasn't cooperating, it was torn out.

"No! No, no, no." Kiko stopped me. "Didn't anybody ever teach you?" I reached into the depths of my earliest memories to recall the moment when someone surely taught me how to properly brush my hair. Among the Rolodex of memories, which includes the time in tenth grade when eleven friends and I all huddled around a single cell phone to receive step-by-step instructions from an upperclassman on how to give head, or the time in first grade when an au pair had taken a fine-toothed comb and eased it through a mayonnaise mask to try to coax the lice out of their homes on my scalp, I could find no memory of being taught me how to properly brush my hair.

Kiko's face was so tender and forgiving, it was as if he had just found an abandoned kitten in a cardboard box. "Like this," he said, and he delicately selected a lock of hair from the forest atop my head and separated it from the rest. Then, beginning at the bottom, not the root, he gently nudged the brush over and over again into the tangle. Nobody had ever paid such careful attention to my hair. Receiving a thoughtful touch like this made me so happy I could've cried. I didn't mean to feel this way, this emotionally moved—I think some spot deep within me was being unexpectedly poked. I received so little *thoughtful touch* when I was young that anytime I get a taste, it feels as exciting as a birthday party with a chocolate fountain. Can you miss something that you never really had? "Here, you try," Kiko told me tenderly, extending the brush. I did my best to imitate his movements. I was not used to being gentle and kind to myself in this way. I was used to getting the thing I wanted through fierce combat rather than tender kindness. I got frustrated with some particularly stubborn knots and reverted back to my trusted technique, but in general, I took to his method. I liked the way it made me feel calm and in control of myself, and I liked how not fighting so hard actually got me closer to my goal. When we were done with brushing, I looked like a kitten but felt like a lion. Then Kiko took over the project entirely. He spun me away from the mirror so I could no longer see myself— this way, the transformation would be more dramatic.

He matted my hair down with a combination of mousse and hair spray. Then he wiped my face clean and covered it with powder. I still wasn't allowed to see myself but I could see the makeup palette Kiko held: an out-of-focus mound of purple dust. He told me with utter confidence that my color was purple and that I should try to wear purple as often as possible.

While hair spray and purple eye shadow are not the first tools I personally reach for when trying to look my best, Kiko had a clear vision for me in a moment when I did not have one for my-self. He put thought into me and that mattered. It made me feel *paid-attention-to*. There are two ways to be paid-attention-to: there is the way where people are judging you, which can make you feel bad, and then there is this way where someone makes you feel special and good. The good kind of attention is filled with what I can only describe as dedication, thoughtfulness, and love. Once we are too old to have a mom or big sister pay atten-tion to us on a daily basis, it is usually up to us to pay attention to ourselves in this loving way. But it is different when the at-tention comes from us versus when it comes from someone else. Both are important. In this moment, Kiko gave all his atten-tion to me. His calmness and confidence jumped from his hands through my hair and into my heart. It made me feel good. Feel-ing good is important. It feels like the start of something great.

When he was done, Kiko held a mirror up so I could get a good look at myself: his creation. I felt like a walking work of art. It wasn't a look I'd wear every day, but this was not every day. This was special. It felt like an encapsulation of my Olympic experience, where I was thrust into an environment that was completely outside of my comfort zone—but it was okay, because I embraced and even celebrated the discomfort. If I had held too tight to the old routines and comforts that I typically rely on before a race, my Olympic experience would have slipped through my fingers like an ice cube. I'm glad I didn't. The purple eye shadow Kiko gave me fucking ruled. I felt ready to face the closing ceremony the next day, like the big dance on the last night of camp. I realized that it was okay to be nervous about the Olympics ending. Nerves are cousin to excitement, and excitement is cousin to gratitude. Pay attention to your nerves: If you feel nervous, it's a sign that a Very Big Thing is unfolding. Be nervous for how good that thing can be.

not your first

not your last

enjoy your *now*

now will go fast

DEPRESSION

When it began, it came in the form of sleeplessness.

I began to lose sleep shortly after returning from Rio. It's not uncommon for Olympians to feel a sort of post-Olympic depression, however mild or severe. It makes sense: You've worked your whole life toward this exceptionally challenging and singular goal, and then it happens, and suddenly it's over. Up until this point, the Olympics are your rising and setting sun. You never think about life after the Olympics because the Olympics themselves can be a life-changer. If you thought about the moment after, you might not get there in the first place. You put everything you have into *getting there*. So when it is over, however well it goes, the feeling is sharp and disorienting. I've spoken with athletes who won gold medals and others who had to drop out of their race, and no matter how someone performed, that post-Olympic "dip" is similar.

I captured that feeling in my movie *Olympic Dreams*—and I've since learned that there's a similar phenomenon in other professions, too. When I met Jimmy Kimmel after my co-star Nick Kroll went on Kimmel's show to promote *Olympic Dreams*, Jimmy told me that he could relate to post-Olympic depression because he also felt a dip after he hosted the Oscars, a professional goal he had worked toward for a long time.

In mild forms, post-Olympic depression is like a ledge. For me, it was a cliff. The entire professional running industry operates in four-year Olympic cycles, where after each Summer Olympics everything gets a reboot. Old contracts expire and new ones are written up. Sometimes entire new teams will form, or athletes and coaches will retire, or athletes will switch sponsors or even change events. It's normal for athletes to check in with themselves and their coach—and their agent, if their endorsement contracts are expiring—after the Olympic cycle ends to make a new plan for the next four years.

The healthy thing to do before planning my next Olympic cycle would have been to take a vacation, or at least a mental break, to give myself time to absorb the enormity of what I had just experienced, and *then* start to plan my next steps with a clear mind and fresh perspective. But instead I felt I needed to keep my momentum going, so when I got back home to Eugene, I continued my training without pause. I would not realize this until much later, but the truth is that for me, I had internalized the idea that being an Olympian would "fix" my deep childhood need to prove to myself that I mattered. But here's the thing about trying to solve an internal problem with an external solution: Even if you achieve the goal you set for yourself, it will never be enough. I desperately wanted to stay one step ahead. Even though I was unsure about what I was really working toward, I felt I just had to *keep working*. I'd never functioned that way before—in the past, when I found myself at a crossroads in life, I always checked in with mentors and with myself to get a full understanding of what my goals were. When

I turned down grad-school scholarships to run at UO, I ana-
lyzed the decision over dinner with my poetry thesis adviser.
When I first started running professionally, I had a vision for
my road to the Olympics. Now I was running blind and feeling
off-balance, not sure exactly what I was training for and why.

On top of that, I was in between creative projects—my creative partner and fiancé, Jeremy, and I had just gotten a distribution deal for our indie film *Tracktown*, so all the work on it
was done. But instead of feeling proud, I felt behind. I immediately put pressure on myself to make a new film even though I
had no idea what our next project would be or how we'd make
it happen. Aside from making it to the Olympics, which was
very much a joint effort, making *Tracktown* had been the North
Star in our lives since graduating from college. Every decision
Jeremy and I made revolved around how we'd pull off making
that movie. Even the decision for me to stay in Eugene after
my fifth year at UO and run for the Nike Oregon Track Club
Elite happened because Jeremy and I had a grand plan to shoot
Tracktown in Eugene. For a significant chunk of our twenties,
everything we did was building to those two huge goals: making
Tracktown and making it to the Olympics. Now that both goals
were behind us, I felt very *in-between*. I felt like my past success
did not guarantee future success and I needed to somehow top
what I already achieved and I needed to have started yesterday.

One of the first things I did back home in Eugene was set up
a call with my agent to discuss my shoe contract. After the
Olympics, my shoe contract with Nike was up for renegotiation.
Even though renegotiating contracts after an Olympic cycle is
normal, the process still made me feel very much in flux at a
vulnerable time. And even though I was now an Olympian,

there was always the chance that my salary could get cut or that I wouldn't get a new offer at all. This often happens in the pro running world, where a sponsor will reduce your contract when they perceive you've reached your peak. Jeremy and I had not yet achieved financial stability as filmmakers, so my shoe contract was a serious matter for us.

Typically, a shoe contract is a runner's primary source of income, and it's also the core tenet of your presence in the professional running world. *Shoe contract* is a bit of a misnomer, as the agreement usually includes apparel as well. For example, if you have a Nike shoe contract, you're obliged to wear Nike shoes and Nike clothes exclusively. Suffice to say, it's easy for an athlete to see their shoe contract as a major part of their identity. When I toed the line in my Nike shoes and Nike uniform, I always felt proud and mighty.

Normally when a shoe contract is up for renegotiation, your agent will "take you to market," meaning he or she will let all the major shoe companies know that you are a free agent. Offers will come in from any companies that are interested, and even if all you want is to re-sign with your previous shoe company, at least now you have some leverage to ensure you're getting a fair deal.

This opportunity to explore the market should have felt like a good thing. But that's not how I saw it at all. Instead I saw it as an unwelcome change being forced on me. Nike felt like family. They had been my sponsor since I entered the pro world. I associated my growth as an Olympic athlete with my relationship with this company. Having my identity wrapped up in a brand was not the healthiest mindset to have: I was irrationally afraid that if I showed any disloyalty to Nike by allowing my agent to communicate with other shoe companies, Nike would not offer to renew my contract. So I instructed my agent to refrain from contacting any other companies, and I even went so far as to personally take a meeting with Nike's head of sports marketing and express my undying loyalty. I was hoping that my performance in Rio and my enthusiasm for the brand would translate into a generous contract. But when Nike's offer came through after months of patient waiting, I was severely disappointed. Compared to the numbers my agent suggested he could have demanded on the open market, this Nike offer was a major undervaluation.

The thing to understand about Nike is that a large part of what they provide exists outside the specific financial scope of the contract, especially if you live in Oregon, where Nike is *everywhere*. As a Nike athlete you have access to training facilities, world-class coaching, elite teammates, and the social cachet of running for a company that everyone knows and admires. This is why athletes often stay with Nike even though they might be getting a smaller compensation package than they would with other companies.

Despite my disappointment at Nike's financial offer, I decided that I could live with it as long as it meant my overall situation was positive and pointing toward my new goals, whatever those would be. So I set a meeting with my coach to get some advice and clarity. I was looking forward to getting direction from him. Coach Ian and I would set goals and life would make sense again.

My expectation was that Ian would encourage me to re-sign with Nike and stay in Eugene with him for another four years, since we had such a good thing going together. But that isn't what happened. Instead, he expressed that this crossroads could be a good opportunity for me to evolve. He told me I was starting to outgrow his small training group of mostly sub-elite boys, and that Eugene might not be the best place for me if I wanted to continue growing athletically. He said I would benefit tremendously from moving up to a bigger-kid playground by training full-time at high altitude in Mammoth Lakes, California, with the Mammoth Track Club elite team. Eugene is one of those places where athletes sometimes overstay their tenure and begin to grow restless. Ian was speaking from experience—he had seen many generations of distance runners, including himself, come through Eugene. It's a great place to grow up, athletically speaking, but at a certain point a long-distance runner needs to graduate to the next level, which, according to Coach Ian, meant living at altitude and joining a new team.

Ian delivered all of this news out of love, of course, but I felt like the rug had been pulled out from under me. I thrive on stability, and more than that, I truly believed in Coach Ian and the life I had built for myself in Oregon. It was working for me and I didn't want to change it. I enjoyed Mammoth Lakes as an altitude training camp, but I had never considered moving there permanently. Even the thought of working with a new coach in a new place with new teammates made me feel sick to my stomach. I didn't have the words to fully express this, but Ian sensed my unease. He explained that he didn't want me to leave Eugene *after* I was ready, he wanted me to leave just before. Eugene had developed me as a college and professional athlete, and Mammoth Lakes would help develop me into a world-class long-distance runner. But I loved Eugene and I loved Ian more than any coach I'd ever had. I didn't understand why this change was needed. I had made it to the Olympics and crushed it, no easy feat. I was basically raised in Eugene, and now it felt like Ian was breaking up with me and making me leave home all at once.

If I had taken some time off and properly recovered after the Olympics, I might have had a healthier perspective. Coach Ian wanted what was best for me and he believed that moving to Mammoth Lakes was how I'd grow as an athlete. Plus, on the film side of my life, Jeremy and I had no real reason to stay in Eugene any longer—*Tracktown* was done and maybe it would be beneficial to both of us to try something new, especially since Mammoth Lakes was much closer to Los Angeles. But in the moment, I couldn't see any of this. All I felt was the blinding anger and fear of someone pushing me out of my home, my nest where I was comfortable.

I am the worst person to push out of a nest. I felt vulnerable and angry. I felt like I was getting left again. An alarm bell that had been gathering dust since my mom died suddenly started ringing again. My rational brain spiraled away down a drain in the back of my mind and fear crawled up to take its place.

With a lump in my gut, I asked my agent to look at what shoe contracts might be out there for me besides Nike. The amount of money Nike offered would not be enough to support me if I moved to Mammoth Lakes, which is a much more expensive place to live and train than Eugene, Oregon. I was afraid I had ruined my chance at finding an offer from a different company, since I had waited so long, but luckily we were able to start a conversation with Under Armour, a company that wanted to make me the new face of their presence in women's running shoes and apparel. Under Armour was prepared to offer me a lot more money than Nike was. I was thrilled and grateful that Under Armour valued me enough to make such a generous offer, but then I tried training in their shoes.

At that time, Under Armour running shoes were unquestionably subpar. Shoes are incredibly important tools for runners, especially when you're running over one hundred miles a week, and lower-quality shoes can lead to injury. I could probably have secretly trained in other shoes and only worn Under Armour shoes to my races and public events, as I heard some of their other sponsored athletes had done, but that left a bad taste in my mouth. Running is as mental as it is physical, and if you show up to a race wearing gear you don't believe in, it will take a toll on your performance. I asked myself: Could I prioritize money over the quality of the shoes?

I thought I needed to force myself to grow up and think more like a businessperson—to prioritize money over my feelings. I would learn, in time, that both matter. It is important to be paid well and it is crucial to believe in the company and products you are representing. I eventually found both in my partnership with Champion, but at the time that opportunity didn't exist yet. At the moment, I could see only what was immediately in front of me: two offers that seemed to be polar opposites, Nike versus Under Armour, with my emotional well-being in one camp and my financial stability in another.

I think I could have handled one of these uncertainties on its own, but grappling with a potential new home, new coach, new team, and new sponsor during this very tenuous post-Olympic time was more than I could bear. I stopped sleeping.

* * *

For some people depression comes on slowly, but for me, it happened all at once. My psychiatrist later described it like this: You are walking along and then suddenly you stumble and fall off a cliff. There is not a perfect equation for what causes someone to get clinical depression. It's highly individual and there are different thresholds for different people. But I wouldn't meet my psychiatrist or understand any of this until much later. All I knew at the moment was that I couldn't sleep. Every night I'd lie in bed, frantically trying to figure out what to do next. It felt like I was brushing my brain with a brush whose bristles were made out of fear and anxiety. I'd rake the brush over my brain again and again, never actually accomplishing anything except depriving myself of sleep until it felt like my whole brain was a knotted tangle of fear.

I felt anxious to do anything I could to climb out of this pit. I feared the worst: Both my mom *and* her brother had died by suicide. That's both kids in her family. As I understand it, their mother—my maternal grandmother—also had struggles with her mental health. With the history of mental illness in my family, I am obligated to tick the box about depression every time I go to the doctor. I am reminded of it constantly. I've always been afraid there is an invisible timer in my head that will one day run out and I will become like my mom, and I was terrified that I was now on a collision course with a destiny that I was desperate to avoid. I thought that if I could handle the situation at hand, I could outrun the darkness that was threatening to engulf me.

My sleeplessness grew worse as nine hours of sleep per night gradually shrank to one, if I was lucky. My mind would not shut off. It felt like my entire *life* was at stake; I was stewing in fear

and anxiety every day. None of these negative feelings came specifically from Nike, Under Armour, my coach, my agent, or
anyone else. They were all deep inside me, attached at their base
to a core of fear that probably has been there since I was little.

It would have been wise to seek help the minute I began having these unhealthy feelings, but that's not what I did. I wasn't
mature enough to see beyond my own fear and resentment
toward change. I wandered circles around the apartment alone,
searching for sleep like buried treasure, but found none. I com-
manded myself to sleep, but we all know that's not how it works.
That's why it's called *falling asleep,* because it's something we let
happen, not make happen. Sleep requires safety, not desperation. My lack of sleep and increasing anxiety were stifling and I
began to have trouble even thinking straight. I was looking at
the world through a kaleidoscope distorted by anxiety and ex-
haustion. The only time I'd feel any respite from my horror
were brief moments of euphoria when I thought about the possibility of going to sleep and never waking up. I was happy because I thought I knew what I needed: to disappear. Knowing
what you need is a nice feeling, except when you're too sick to
think.

I tried to put on a brave face and embrace change as growth.
Even though I was in no position mentally to be making such
big life decisions, I signed the Under Armour term sheet and
made arrangements with the Mammoth Track Club to join the
team full-time. I should have asked for a fully executed countersigned contract with Under Armour before I moved to Mammoth Lakes, as my agent suggested, but I wasn't thinking
logically and I just wanted to keep moving forward, like a shark

that never stops swimming, not even in its sleep. Jeremy and I gave our Eugene landlords notice and found a new place in Mammoth Lakes. We drove down together and then I settled in to train while Jeremy went back to Eugene to pack up our old house. But even though my actions indicated that I was making progress, inside I was regressing into a mental place I'd never been before. All I wanted to do was curl up in a ball and go back in time to the way things were before. I felt like I was losing my grip on reality. I was always so good at planning my life and working hard to achieve the goals I set, no matter how lofty, but now I was in a complete free fall.

The only healthy thing I could have done at that point would have been to stop everything and get help. But instead I continued to train as hard as ever in Mammoth Lakes, running up to 120 miles a week at 8,000 feet on one hour of sleep per night. That kind of mileage is hard with ten hours of sleep and a nap every day, as I always had done when I took training trips to Mammoth Lakes in the past. You can't run that much mileage without recovering, and sleep is the most important means for the body to bounce back from that level of strain without getting injured.

There was no doubt that my body was breaking down just like my mind. My stress level kept climbing. I later learned that the mind is more susceptible to depression at higher altitudes. The combination of anxiety and sleeplessness was the worst feeling I've ever had, like an invisible searing hot pan. It was untouchable. Sleeplessness turned me into a different person. It didn't allow my brain and body and heart to be on the same page. And when your brain and body and heart are on different pages it tears you apart like tissue paper. I was so bleary-eyed that I couldn't even see myself anymore. I was a running zombie.

I didn't slow down. If anything I only sped up and tried to run through it. I trained harder. I tried to continue pushing forward even though something was obviously not right. I didn't ask for help and I even rejected it, despite being gripped by agonizing anxiety and uncertainty every day. As a result, I mishandled my first few conversations with my new team at Under Armour. Instead of being charming and collaborative, I was undiplomatic. The marketing person in charge of my contract was aware that I had concerns about Under Armour's running shoes, and she set up a meeting with the shoe design team for me to give feedback. I had legitimate questions and suggestions about their plans for a line of quality training and racing shoes, which even they acknowledged was underdeveloped compared to other companies, but I worded my thoughts in a fearful and aggressive way. I wasn't wrong about the facts—they had no plans to invest energy or resources into developing their high-end running shoes at that time—but I was so strung out from lack of sleep that I spoke with absolutely no filter. I can imagine that I came across as combative and difficult.

After that meeting, Under Armour rescinded my contract and pulled their offer. Since they had not countersigned and fully executed the contract, they were legally within their rights to leave. I beat myself up endlessly and blamed myself for all of this. When you are depressed, everything feels like it's your fault. And while I do wish I had carried myself with more grace during my brief time at Under Armour, I know now that the partnership would have felt hollow without everyone agreeing about what matters most from a shoe contract: quality running shoes.

In the meantime, my previous offer from Nike had expired. I was left with nothing and it was looking like I'd be without an income. In the midst of my extreme anxiety I continued to train hard without sleeping and, sure enough, I developed the first serious injury of my life. As an athlete, it was remarkable that I had not gotten a single injury until then, at age twenty-seven. My injury was clearly stress related, a partial hamstring tear, easy to develop if you sleep one hour a night and train like an Olympian. Unfortunately, Mammoth Lakes is such a small town that the medical resources were limited. There were no physical therapists available who had experience working with Olympic-level distance runners.

I had an ominous feeling that I had somehow irreparably jeopardized my ability to be a professional athlete. I was convinced that if I could only *go back* and reverse the events of the past few months, I could fix everything. I tried to undo everything I'd done, which should have been another sign I needed help. The minute you start looking backward, when you entertain the idea of trying to unscramble an egg, you need to ask for help. You need to stop moving and deal with yourself at exactly where you are in that moment.

But rather than stop and evaluate, I made fast, flailing moves to save what I saw as my rapidly sinking career. I probably could have corrected course, stopped training to let my hamstring heal, and salvaged my contract opportunity—but depression can distort how you see yourself and your place in the world. I thought I needed to be in my old town, with my old coach and my old trainers, running my old trails with my old teammates, sponsored by my old brand. I wanted my old everything.

Jeremy had just finished packing up our old house in Oregon and was literally on the road in a U-Haul halfway between Eugene and Mammoth Lakes—a thirteen-hour drive—when I called him and told him to turn around and go back to Eugene because I wasn't sure that we could survive in Mammoth Lakes anymore. I told him I would meet him there. Bewildered, Jeremy drove the truck all the way back to Eugene and spent the night on a sleeping bag in our empty house because we had one night left in our lease, and then we crashed with friends, not knowing how long we would be there. All of our belongings were now spread among our condo in Mammoth Lakes, a storage unit in Eugene, and the suitcase we kept at whichever friend's place where we were crashing. One week in Eugene became two, became three, became I can't even remember how long, while Jeremy and I bounced between friends' couches, Airbnbs, and house-sitting gigs.

Shortly after our retreat back to Eugene, I left town to accompany my old teammates to training camp in Flagstaff, Arizona. Even though I was injured and even though I wasn't on that team anymore, I still insisted on going to the training camp. I wasn't even able to train but I stubbornly wanted to be there anyway. At some point during the camp it was my birthday, and I was so sad and miserable that I didn't tell anyone. My teammates and I went to Chipotle for dinner and I was so out of it that I asked the cashier if my burrito would be free since it was my birthday. That's how my teammates found out it was my birthday. They felt bad but I felt worse.

From Flagstaff, I flew to Chicago to make an appearance at the Shamrock Shuffle 8k race, a commitment that had been made months prior. I was the reigning champion of the Shamrock Shuffle, having won the race for the past two years in a row, but now I felt like a shell of that person. I was depressed, but even worse, I was injured and unable to race. As an athlete, I found it impossible to separate my identity from my injured body.

Even though I was in no position to be traveling or making a public appearance, I insisted on honoring my commitment to go to the Shamrock Shuffle because I was too proud and stubborn to admit anything was wrong. I felt like I was trying to catch all the feathers bursting from a torn pillow. The race directors in Chicago knew I was injured and couldn't *race* the thing, but I told them I could still run it slower with one of their investors. I was desperate not to drop out of this event because I felt I needed to continue to do everything I was supposed to be doing. *Supposed to* was another phrase I couldn't let go of—I was supposed to do this and I was supposed to be that—so I kept doing things that helped me appear normal to the outside world, but none of which would help me heal myself. I ended up jogging the race with a little girl who looked up to me and I tried my best to be there for her during a time when I was not being there for myself. Despite being completely terrified inside and also in severe physical pain, I managed to pull it off. There are articles written about me being a role model that day, and while I am proud to have been a positive presence at the race, it scares me to think about how well I was able to cover up what was really going on inside.

People did not understand what was going on inside my

mom's head, either, when she started to lose it. I have been told that nobody knew the extent to which she was sick. We are both brilliant smilers and perpetual overachievers, and as I understand it, my mom tried until she died. She pretended everything was okay when it wasn't. And now here I was, doing the exact same thing.

I remember swimming in the pool at the Hilton in Chicago after the race, and I floated on my back and thought about how I'd screwed up my life in a way that I never thought possible. I felt *doom*. That was a new feeling for me, the sinking feeling that things are irreversibly bad and will never get better. I wanted to drown.

Floating in the pool and staring into nowhere, I realized that my worst nightmare was coming true: I reminded myself of my mother. I could feel her calling to me the way the sirens called to Odysseus. I thought back to the old photo album that contains the only pictures I have of her. It's from sometime during her high-school years: Some of the photos are from her sweet sixteen, others are of former boyfriends, some are from school choir performances and baseball games, and a few are from graduation. She was successful, beautiful, and popular. Whenever I looked at the photo album, I felt weird that the smiling girl in the pictures didn't know that she'd one day take her own life. How could she be so happy in this moment and then become something else entirely? When did the switch happen, and could she see it coming?

For my whole life I'd prided myself on how different from my mother I was. I was quite certain that I was above it all, that what happened to her could not happen to me. I had to see myself as different from her for my own survival. But when I thought about seeing her look so genuinely happy as a teenager in the photo album, it scared me. It reminded me of all the photos of myself smiling at the Olympics. I had no idea that just a few months after those photos were taken, my entire life would feel like it was falling apart.

People have told me they did everything they could to help my mom but she was unable to be helped. I started to worry that like her, I was *un-helpable*. When I was younger, I had sympathy for my mother—how sad she must have been! But now I felt *empathy* for her. This is the strongest connection I've ever felt to my mom: when I finally understood what it felt like to want to disappear.

I never wanted to get to know her in this way. I never wanted to actually feel anything approaching what she must have felt. I used to think about all the ways I wanted to live, and now I thought about all the ways I could die. It was so sad, the saddest feeling I've ever experienced. At the same time, this type of understanding is something I think I've craved my whole life. I grew up feeling like everyone else in the world knew my mother better than me: her friends, her teachers, my dad, my brother—everyone. People who knew her would often try to tell me about her—your mom was a good athlete, your mom used to sew—and while I liked learning things about her, it also reminded me how much I didn't know her. But now, in this fucked-up way, I understood her more than anyone else could.

* * *

Growing up, I had no problem asking for help. I spent my whole life unashamedly latching on to mentors and seeking out their expertise. But in those cases, I only felt unknowledgeable or confused, not *crazy*. I'd always been the successful person asking for guidance, not the unstable person asking for rescue. It is hard for a successful person to ask for help in that way. It's dangerous when you decide you must always be "okay" because everyone thinks you are and that's all they've ever known of you. Sometimes the strongest, most successful people haven't developed the muscle that knows when and how to ask for the help they need.

When I got back from Chicago, my former UO teammate and roommate Anne was visiting Eugene from Germany. She had come all the way from Europe and had five precious days to visit the place where she felt most at home, the place where so many of us found our potential and grew into ourselves. When Anne and I met up, it was immediately clear to her that something was terribly wrong with me. I was able to fake it during my public appearances, but it is hard to fake it with good friends. We went on a walk in the woods where we used to run and I wasn't even able to talk to her in full sentences. I kept stuttering and then eventually crying. Anne was never one to freak out. It was her calmness that, way back when, helped our team win a National Championship title. I remember Anne calming me down the night before the race—assuring me that I would not let everyone down, as I feared. She told me I would be okay, because she knew I would be.

But this time, Anne wasn't sure if I was okay. I told her I had ruined my career. I told her I wasn't sleeping. I told her I was injured. I told her that everything was hopeless and that I wished I could go back in time. I told her that I'd walk to the grocery store way more than I needed to and just wander around without buying anything. I didn't tell her that every time I heard a train whistle—trains often passed through Eugene—I'd think about lying on the tracks. The train whistle felt like it was beckoning me. After our walk ended, Anne didn't want to let me be alone. Instead she called Kimber, another friend and former UO teammate. Even though Anne only had five days to visit Eugene, she and Kimber decided to arrange a mini-trip to Portland to go wedding-dress shopping. My wedding was coming up in just a few months—Jeremy and I had started planning our wedding and even sent out "save the dates" a few weeks before all the insanity began—and now, in my depression, wedding-dress shopping was not something I could wrap my mind around. Anne and Kimber merrily but calmly drove me the two hours to Portland and ignored my repeated apologies for how much of a downer I was being. They didn't make me feel weird for feeling weird.

When we got to Portland I told them I didn't feel like trying on dresses anymore and asked if we could just drive the two hours back to Eugene, but they persisted, patiently. Anne and Kimber are just the right amount of stubborn, the amount that you need in your life when you are severely depressed, especially when you don't yet understand that you are severely depressed. I didn't need them to tell me I was crazy or pathetic, I could already feel that myself. And I didn't need them to push me away and tell me to get help, I wasn't ready for that yet. I needed them to let me cry in the car, then buy me a cold-pressed juice, wipe my face, and get my ass into the Anthropologie fitting room. Friends help you feel dignified even when you do not. Like when I fell in the steeplechase water pit during a practice run the day before a huge race, and Anne jumped in with me just to save me from being embarrassed in front of the rival team's coach, who made a snide comment when he saw me fall. "There, now we're both wet," she said triumphantly. Humiliation cannot survive when a friend is by your side.

At Anthropologie, I actually ended up finding the skirt I wore to my wedding. The pictures of me trying on the skirt are miserable—I look like what I imagine Sylvia Plath would look like in a wedding gown. I have a photo where I am wearing a gown while holding the complimentary glass of champagne they give you, with a backdrop of other brides-to-be, and I look heartbreakingly sad, like a wilting rose. Now I love that photo because it's a reminder of how good my friends were to me during this terrible time, and when my wedding day eventually came, I was so happy to have that skirt. That's kind of how getting help is when you're in denial about being sick: You don't want it in the moment, but eventually you will be happy you got it.

Shortly after the shopping trip, even though I hadn't yet spoken the words and admitted that I was depressed and needed serious help, Jeremy and I decided to postpone our wedding. We both knew we were in no place to plan a wedding. How could we? Our lives were completely derailed. Jeremy was still busy with managing *Tracktown* from afar, helping the distributors get all the materials ready for the release, but he was in flux just as much as I was—our lives and careers were completely intertwined. We didn't know where we'd be sleeping any given week and we had no stable income. Composing that email to our guests explaining why we were delaying our wedding was quite a task: We didn't want to reveal too much and alarm anyone, but we also needed to tactfully justify changing our wedding date after many people had already made travel plans. It wasn't pleasant, but it was necessary.

Shortly after we pushed back the wedding date, Jeremy's parents came out to visit us in Eugene. I took a walk in the woods with his mom on my favorite trail ever, a gorgeous winding path through Hendricks Park, but I was not even able to enjoy the misty wet leaves of Eugene flopping lazily over their moss-covered branches. In the past, whenever I was feeling down, a run through Hendricks Park would always leave me feeling better. Trail running in the woods is one of my favorite activities. It gives me a different type of joy than road running or racing; it's a joy that touches every sense individually and makes me feel ebullient, present, and connected to the earth. But not this time. I was weary, like a used tea bag, unable to appreciate ordinary wonderful things. And it was getting worse. Still, I did not ask for help.

Several weeks had passed since Jeremy and I retreated from Mammoth Lakes and started couch-hopping in Eugene. Moving from one friend's house to the next was wearing on everybody and it was getting to the point where we needed to commit to staying in Eugene and find a place of our own or commit to fully moving to Mammoth Lakes. But we weren't ready to make a decision like that. That decision rested largely on my running career, and I could hardly get out of bed in the morning, let alone decide where I wanted to train. Thankfully, salvation came in the form of one of the most wonderful professional runners I know, Andy Wheating. Andy owned a large house in the hills of Eugene, which he had just listed for sale. Like me, Andy was making a post-Olympic life change. His roommates had cleared out and the house was spotless, but Andy graciously let

Jeremy and me stay in the second bedroom until we could get on our feet, or until the house sold. I think Andy had an idea of what was going on, but, like Anne, he never made me feel bad about it. I am so grateful to him for the shelter—literal and figurative. I think there is a wonderful understanding between professional athletes that some moments are harder than others. Thanks to Andy, Jeremy and I had a stable yet not permanent place to stay. It was exactly what we needed in that moment.

With a bit more stability, I tried to get back into a routine in Eugene that somewhat approached the normal life I remembered. It didn't exactly feel like things were getting better, but at least I didn't feel like I was in free fall anymore. I felt comfortably settled at rock bottom. I was living a ghost version of my old life. I was injured, without a shoe contract, and had no particular goal, but at least I knew where I was sleeping for the foreseeable future. Every day felt like a haze and I accepted as fact that my life as I knew it was over, irreparably damaged, and now it was my fate to exist in perpetual misery.

* * *

Throughout all of this, my dad called regularly to make sure I was okay. Over the weeks and months since the Olympics ended, he had been there for countless phone calls where I described step by step the unfolding disaster that was my life. He has always been super calm and there to listen to me, rock-solid and attentive, but never stepping in to save me. He lets me fail and succeed on my own. My dad understands that it is natural and normal for children to struggle and that it's not always productive for a parent to intervene.

But this time was different. He was hearing things that were red flags. Things that might have reminded him of my mother. Unlike Jeremy, who was right there in the thick of it with me, my dad could see from afar that something wasn't right. Sometimes it takes a certain kind of distance from a situation to see it clearly, like how you can't stand too close to a Seurat painting and understand what it is. My brother was also concerned for me. Our family has always functioned more like a team than a typical family hierarchy, so when something is wrong, we all know. For the first time, my dad told me I needed *professional help*. He wasn't willing to be a patient ear any longer—he had heard enough and was putting his foot down. I needed to see a doctor.

My dad hardly ever puts his foot down, so when he does, I listen. There's no use in *not* listening—he's just too stubborn. Plus, he's almost always right, and this sort of mandate from him was so rare that I knew it warranted attention.

At first, like many people who need help, I was defensive. Psychiatric help can feel scary and unnecessarily extreme. Up until this point, the last time I'd spoken to a mental health professional was shortly after my mom died, and I hated how the "talking doctor," as we called him, would watch me play with toys and ask me questions, and then tell my dad everything I had said, like a tattletale. But despite my pushback against seeing a doctor, my dad and brother were persistent and any time I spoke with either one of them, they demanded I get help. I am stubborn, but in my heart I always trust my family. So finally I relented and told them that I'd try. All my dad has ever asked of me is that I try.

The first thing I did was to reach out to a life coach in South

Carolina named Gayle. Jeremy's family knew Gayle and it seemed like a good fit. In my mind it felt better to work with a life coach than a "talking doctor." But a life coach is not a trained professional doctor who can handle someone who is sick. A life coach is helpful for people who are swerving within their lane, not for people who have veered off the road entirely.

Gayle and I first talked over Skype, and right away I knew that talking with her wasn't going to really help me. To be honest, it felt hard for me to talk to a woman about my feelings. It was usually my dad, my brother, or Jeremy who helped me in times of crisis. As a result, I didn't feel comfortable with her feminine energy and emotional approach to talking about my situation. It's not that I don't look up to women—there are so many women I look up to—but I either do or I don't. I know this isn't the best thing to admit, but it's my truth. I'm never sure if, when I open up to a woman, it will help me or humiliate me.

Gayle told me things like "Love yourself!," but I didn't know how to love myself. She told me to get away. Go anywhere! The beach! A vacation! This turned out not to be what I needed. When you are depressed and spinning out, escaping is not the answer. You don't need to get away, you need to stay put. But instead I listened to Gayle. Jeremy and I tried to go to the Oregon coast one weekend, but he got frustrated and chastised me the entire drive there for not being happy. He didn't understand that depression was not a choice—he said he missed the old me and asked if I could just be myself again, otherwise he wasn't sure if he could keep being with me. It was an impossible demand and it broke my heart. To someone who is clinically depressed, being told to "just be yourself again" or being reminded that "your life is really good" is very difficult and counterproductive. Hearing those things made me feel worse; it made me feel spoiled and damaged beyond repair because I could not force myself to appreciate the good things in my life, and just *be myself* again. It's hard to have gratitude when you're depressed.

My mom also felt pressure from her family to "snap out of it." My dad recently showed me a letter that my mom's mom sent in 1994, just a few months before my mother killed herself—it's a miracle he still has any of her old letters at all, he found it at the bottom of a box of old paperwork when he was cleaning out his garage. The words my grandmother wrote felt all too familiar:

> I'm not going to give you a lecture—Robbie—I want to let you know—<u>I love you</u>—<u>but cannot</u> understand you at this time. Nobody is going to help you <u>now</u> except <u>you</u> yourself—and since you <u>have so much</u> to live for—try harder.
>
> We, most women, have to give up things—if they want a Home + family—you must learn to be <u>responsible</u> for the things you choose to <u>do</u>. I would do it all over again—what a pleasure it is to see a child develop into a person—give you the love you give to them. Enjoy it—because it all goes so quickly. Can't believe I'm so old already and how lucky I am to have made it with my husband + my children + grandchildren. Many people are NOT that lucky. Glad I can get out of bed + try to enjoy every day + <u>be thankful with what I have.</u>
>
> I will write to you—if you write—I will talk to you <u>only</u> when you <u>Honestly</u> tell me you are <u>well</u>. Decided—you are the only <u>one</u> who can shape your

life (or destiny) and make yourself better. Try
Harder.
    Kiss the kids for me. Only want to hear Good
News from you Robbie.
    Always, Mom

This letter makes me so sad. My grandmother thought she was helping my mom. But I know from experience that a letter like this would not have helped. It would have hurt, very badly. Maybe she was a product of her time, but my grandmother did not understand or acknowledge depression as a mental illness. She saw it as a *choice* and she didn't want anything to do with it. This is why my grandmother didn't go to my mom's funeral, because she never accepted that my mom was sick in the first place.

On the Oregon coast with Jeremy, all I wanted to do was jump off the jagged cliffs and die in the ocean. I thought everything and everyone would be better off that way. To be suicidal is to live in a perpetual "grass is greener" state of mind, where you're convinced by the illusion that everything you are not is better than what you are, including being alive.

Talking to Gayle, the life coach, made my situation seem simpler than it was, as if I could change my feelings by telling myself to feel something else. But no matter how hard I tried I couldn't succeed in changing my feelings, which, in turn, made me feel worse. I would later learn that it's actually quite hard to tell yourself to change your feelings, even when you're completely healthy. You have to change your actions, then your thoughts and feelings will follow. But I did not understand this yet. Instead, I felt increasingly inadequate that I couldn't translate what Gayle told me into making myself feel any better, like I was not even capable of being helped. I felt useless, and therefore I felt worthless.

Meanwhile, I was trying to heal my hamstring injury by going to at least two appointments a day with massage therapists, acupuncturists, doctors, and physiotherapists, none of whom seemed to be able to help. My days were spent bouncing from one appointment to the next—I saw any doctor who could fit me in and I said yes to anything that would have even a remote chance of helping. One doctor gave me cortisone shots, another administered a painful pelvic floor exam (administered by palpating my pelvic floor through my vagina), and another physical therapist did so much dry needling to my leg that an MRI showed I had significant internal hemorrhaging. Some of the doctors told me I'd never run again. It was confusing, invasive, disheartening, and irresponsible. It was not smart or effective to be seeking out every form of help that could possibly exist and embracing every doctor's suggestion; I was not mentally fit enough to be responsible for my physical care. I couldn't be calm, I couldn't sit still, I couldn't think about anything but doom.

I was also trying to salvage my contract with Nike. After I wrote a pleading email to the head of the sports marketing division, I was offered a revised version of my prior contract with an even lower financial package than before. It wasn't enough money to live on, but in a dazed panic, I signed it.

One week later, with increasing insistence from my dad and brother, I finally agreed to see a psychiatrist. It was clear that my situation was more serious than something I could talk through with a life coach. I tried to make an appointment but every psychiatrist seemed to be booked indefinitely. I was learning how hard it can be to get the help you need when you finally understand that you need it. At last, through a personal referral, I got an appointment with two different psychiatrists so I could make sure I found one who worked for me. The first one I met with was a stern woman who reminded me of the helicopter mom I never had. She wore a bright red pantsuit with her hair pulled back tight. She asked me very stern, detailed questions about my thoughts. She listened to my symptoms and then looked at me how a mom might look at her kids if she caught them trying to pierce their own ears, and immediately told me that she was afraid I was going to kill myself *any day now*. The horrified way she looked at me was how *I* began to look at me. When you're depressed you become like a sponge, soaking in everything around you no matter what it is.

She raised her voice. She said she'd never met someone like me—usually a good thing, except in this case. She said I was an extremely high-risk case—she called me a *case*, not a person—and said that I needed to get on the highest dose of the strongest antidepressant as soon as possible. She wanted to put me on medication that would sedate me entirely so that I would not have the will to kill myself if my suicidal thoughts got any worse. This kind of medication also takes away your will to do anything and effectively turns you into a walking potato. She told me I would need to find a psychologist separately, because she was a psychiatrist. She would prescribe medicine and a psychologist would focus more on talk therapy—usually, she explained, you work with both in tandem. I was daunted by the idea of navigating two different doctors, one for medication and one for therapy. I left the appointment feeling even more like a failure.

Then I met with Dr. Arpaia, who, along with my dad, saved my life. Dr. Arpaia was both a psychiatrist and a psychologist, specializing in cognitive behavioral therapy. He wore giant T-shirts with wild animals on them, the kind you see for sale at gas stations. He had kind eyes. He didn't raise his voice. I felt calm around him. Like with a coach, it is very important to find a healthcare professional you believe in. I told Dr. Arpaia what was going on in my life—the contracts, the move, everything. I also told him how you only get one chance at everything in life and I had messed it up. It was all my fault and I was so spoiled and stupid to think I deserved more than I was being offered, and I was especially stupid for not being grateful for what I had before and thinking I could survive in a new place. I told him that if I could only go back in time I could fix things, but since that was impossible I had accepted that I'd had a good life, but my bubble of good luck had run out and there was no way out of the mess I had created. My life would never be better than it was before and frankly, it would be better to die now because my best days were behind me, and it's better to quit when you're ahead. I had been thinking these things in a repetitive, taunting way, like a soundtrack incessantly playing in my head. There was almost a hubris to my depression, where I felt worthless but at the same time my mind assumed it could predict the future. Depression is more than just sadness; it's an entire distortion of perspective. I was feeling the lowest feelings a person can ever feel.

Admitting all of this to Dr. Arpaia, still a stranger to me, was hard but also easy. It can be easier to admit the embarrassing things to someone who doesn't know you. He listened quietly, much like my dad might have, and calmly explained to me that I was sick. He told me I was experiencing an *acute crisis*—high-risk situational depression—which is when everything is going great and then suddenly, specific things occur in your life that make you feel like you've fallen off a cliff. This was the first time I'd been given a diagnosis that I understood.

Oh my god. I was sick. I was sick. I was sick. I was *mentally ill*. It was temporary, but it was severe. It was the realest worst thing I could ever imagine. But at the same time it was so unbelievably refreshing to meet someone who understood exactly what was going on. He explained that mental illness is like when you fall and have a scrape on your knee—except instead of the cut being on your knee, it is on your brain. It takes time to heal. Your brain is a body part that can get injured like any other, and it can also heal like any other. My hamstring injury started out as a sore leg that I could have fixed on my own with some rest. As the soreness got worse, my leg probably just needed a good physio or massage therapist. But eventually, the sore leg turned into a torn tendon that needed medical intervention because it could no longer heal on its own. When you tear a tendon, you need a doctor. The rest and physical therapy that *would have* healed you earlier simply isn't enough anymore.

My brain was the same way. What began as post-Olympic depression could have probably been okay if I had taken some time to rest and mentally recover. When I started feeling anxiety and fear after Coach Ian recommended I leave Eugene, a life coach could have helped me get perspective and overcome my negative thoughts. But after months of living in a perpetual state of fight-or-flight mode, I had a "tear" in my mind that needed professional help just like the tear in my tendon. My brain was chemically altered and needed medical intervention. I think many people make the same mistake of not taking a mental injury as seriously as they would a physical injury. This is probably because a mental injury is invisible and doesn't necessarily limit you from showing up to work or otherwise continuing your regular routine, however terrible it might feel inside.

There's a reason why professionals exist, in every form. Dr. Arpaia told me he would not put me on severe medication because he didn't want to drug me out of this. He would pair medication (mild antidepressants and pills to help me fall asleep) with intensive talk therapy. The medication was necessary to jump-start my mind into healing itself, but medication is never enough on its own—it needs to be paired with talk therapy so that as the medication helps your brain return to a normal chemical balance, you are taking advantage of that physical healing to work on emotional healing.

I did not believe I could ever emerge from my depression happier than I was before, but I had nothing to lose. I already wanted to die, so why not give this a try? Why not live one more day and see what happens? That mantra got me through so many days—the thought that things couldn't possibly get any worse, so they could only get better. Even though I was convinced they *wouldn't* get better, I could live another day, and another, and another, just to see. It was like watching my own experiment of myself. Dr. Arpaia understood why I felt this way and he didn't make me feel bad about it. Actually, he told me I was doing great, even though I did not feel great. He gave me one of the most valuable truths anyone has ever taught me: First your *actions* change, then your *thoughts*, then finally your *feelings*, in that specific order. He told me to stop trying to convince myself to not be depressed—a depressed person can't be convinced of anything. He told me to instead expect that I was going to feel very sad for a long time, and that the most important thing was to focus on my actions. Actions change your thoughts over time, and over even more time thoughts change your feelings.

It's sort of like when you are in a race and you might feel absolutely terrible in one moment, but that doesn't mean you should stop. In a race I never rely solely on how I feel in a moment—because it will almost always be the case that I'm hurting, and it's also almost always the case that I can push through a rough patch of pain. Racing is very painful, but we are not what we feel in any single moment and just because I'm in the hurt box now doesn't mean I won't feel better in a few more laps. Racing is about understanding that pain is a sensation but not necessarily a threat, and if you continue to put one foot in front of the other you *will* break through your rough patch.

Likewise, I now understood that my mental rough patch could be handled similarly by showing up one day at a time and putting in the work with Dr. Arpaia to get my life back on track. I needed to take myself forward with actions like you might take a crying toddler through a grocery store: You still need to get the milk even if the toddler is crying. I stopped judging or even thinking about my bleak feelings and dark thoughts. I had faith that if I focused on my actions—on going to therapy, rehabbing my injury, and making a plan for the future—my feelings would get better in time. This new understanding saved my life.

* * *

I promised myself I would become dedicated to curing my depression as if it were my next Olympics. Healing my brain was even more important than healing my hamstring. This is something my dad helped me understand. He told me that taking care of my brain was the most essential thing in the world. He told me that it might be the hardest thing I ever did but that it'd be worth it. He told me to trust him and I did. He told me to promise him I'd keep showing up—as always, my dad told me to try. For the first time in my life, I prioritized self-care and maintenance over productivity and performance.

There were moments when I wanted to give up, probably ten times a day. When those moments came, I called my dad, who always picked up the phone. I cannot thank him enough for always answering the fucking phone—no matter what. I would try to go on a run and not be able to run more than a mile without stopping to walk and to cry. Everything around me that used to make me happy—the trees, the smells, the sky—now made me sad. I felt like an *other* in a world I used to know and love. During these times, I'd call my dad and he was always the one to hang up the phone last.

I told him things I never thought I'd admit, not even to myself. Mind you, I never even told my dad when I had boyfriends growing up, and in my early teenage years I preferred to cut my underwear into homemade thongs rather than ask him to take me panty shopping, so to now share that I was having thoughts about dying was really hard. I would tell him I wanted to die almost every day. I had obsessive thoughts of wanting to die. But he knew that I was calling him because I didn't actually *want to* want to die. There is a big difference. He told me "Keep going, Lex," like he always did. He said I could do anything in the world except quit. He told me to just keep going. He asked me to do it for him. This was one of the only times I've ever heard my dad cry. He told me we weren't going to lose this time, and I knew exactly what he meant.

Even if my own heart was broken, I wasn't going to break his. I would show up every day and do whatever I was told. Dr. Arpaia became my new coach. I saw him three times a week and he gave me exercises ranging from going for a walk, to breathing techniques, to visualization exercises to help me fall asleep. Any time I tried to lie down I'd inevitably start thinking about something I had done wrong and then a cascade of dreadful thoughts would overwhelm me. Dr. Arpaia told me to conjure an image that was completely disassociated from my life and fixate my mind's eye on that until sleep took me. My favorite thing to visualize was an image of myself curled up inside a walnut shell, completely cozy and protected from the outside world.

Dr. Arpaia also gave me a notebook and he'd have me write down certain things over and over again, like when I had to write "Day by day, in every way, I'm getting better and better" one hundred times. Another day my assignment was to write "I have a body but I'm not my body, I have thoughts but I am not my thoughts, I have feelings but I am not my feelings." And another day I had to write all the things I was mad at myself for and then forgive myself, like: "I forgive you for the contract," or "I forgive you for being injured," or "I forgive you for being mean to your dad," and then finish it with "and I love you any-way."

Dr. Arpaia didn't make me feel bad if one exercise didn't res-onate with me. He gave me another piece of advice: Find what's useful and focus on that. Focus only on what's useful.

This advice became particularly resonant to me when I started to have epically fantastic dreams, and then I would wake up and the real world was a nightmare. In the best dream I ever had, Sarah Silverman was in my high-school Spanish class and she gave me a stuffed owl, which I understood was an official invitation to audition for *Saturday Night Live*. When I woke up I was so happy about the dream, but then suddenly so sad in real life. The better the dreams, the worse real life felt afterward. I told Dr. Arpaia that I never wanted to wake up because my dreams were so good and real life was so bad, and he told me, fine, to start taking my dreams more seriously, then. Sure, they were dreams, but they made me happy—he told me that this was my mind's way of trying to slowly help me, and that if it was useful, to pretend my dreams were real. It was helpful to under-stand that anything that helped me feel good, no matter how unexpected the source, was okay. As long as it's not harmful, everything is fair game when you're trying to survive depres-sion. It was also lovely to believe that, deep inside, by creating good dreams, I was subconsciously trying to help myself.

Focusing on what's useful also applied to people. This was fucking survival and I needed to get myself out of this hole, so I didn't share with very many people what was going on. It takes a lot of energy to share, and in this moment, I needed all the energy I could muster just to make it to the next day. Dr. Arpaia urged me to share my experiences only with people who were useful to me: Jeremy, and my dad, and my brother. Very few other people had any idea of what kind of intense treatment I was undergoing, and this was extremely important. The energy I put into healing myself was tremendous and there was none to spare for updating friends or otherwise opening up to other people. I didn't want attention, I wanted to *heal*. Healing was the hardest thing I've ever done, and I've done some hard things. Writing this book is the first time I've spoken openly about what I went through, and I suspect many of my friends will learn about it for the first time by reading these pages.

My work with Dr. Arpaia continued for five months. I was sad almost every day. And I mean really, really sad. But you can be sad and motivated at the same time. I kept reminding myself that actions change first, then thoughts, then feelings. Viewing the present from the future is very difficult but worth it. It's like running a painful race: It takes gritty persistence to keep putting one foot in front of the other, but you can handle the pain because you expect there will be a future you who crosses the finish line. Likewise, when you expect sadness every day, but also know that you are taking the actions you need to in order to improve, the sadness becomes more manageable. I stopped judging my sadness and focused only on my actions. I brought the same relentless dedication that I'd normally bring to my athletic training to my mental recovery. I kept taking my medicine, completing the exercises Dr. Arpaia gave me, and trying to slowly progress in the other areas of my life.

In the middle of my recovery, I had to give a speech to a running club in Grapevine, Texas. I was afraid of repeating my experience at the Shamrock Shuffle in Chicago, where everyone looked at me as a role model even though I felt so sad. I thought about not going to Texas, but Dr. Arpaia and I decided together that I could do it. He helped me prepare for the visit. When I got there, I did a run with a crowd of high-school kids and had a slip in mental strength. I felt like an imposter. It reminded me of the scene in the movie *Big Fish,* where the main character finds himself in Specter, a surreal town where everyone is permanently happy. I felt paranoid: Why were people looking up to me? I was not worth looking up to. Dr. Arpaia helped me understand that this was not true, that I belonged there despite my sadness. He told me all of this in texts and on phone calls he took throughout the weekend, for which I am very grateful.

The difference between this appearance in Texas and my visit to Chicago was that Dr. Arpaia helped me see myself from a bird's-eye view: I understood that I was depressed, and so I *expected* to feel sadness—and just like I could prepare myself to manage pain during a race, now I could prepare myself to manage sadness. So when I felt the sadness come on, I focused on my actions and continued with my job. That night there was a banquet and I gave the closing speech. People hung on my every word. It went well. Of course I still felt weird inside, like I didn't belong there, like I didn't deserve to be standing in my own shoes. But I ignored those thoughts as best I could.

After the speech, a group of teenage girls came up to me and asked for my autograph. It meant a lot to me. It reminded me of the time when my family had dinner at a tiny Italian restaurant in Malibu, and sitting across the dining room from us was Robert Downey, Jr. I was six years old and didn't know who he was, but since I was the youngest and cutest of the group, my dad's friend urged me to go say hi and ask for his autograph. He had recently gotten out of jail. In fact, he looked like he had just left jail that day. I remember he seemed so sad, taking bites of his pasta. But I still went up to him and asked for his autograph. I wasn't sure how he'd react, but then he looked me in the eye and said, "Little girl, you just made my night." I doubt he remembers this but I will never forget it. And I never understood quite how I made his night until that night in Grapevine when those girls asked for my autograph. Sometimes, it's when you feel least powerful that you can be touched the deepest. Those girls saw me how I wanted to see myself.

Slowly, I began to heal. I was sad, deeply sad, for at least six months. But sure enough, the sadness began to slip away, like I was a snake shedding its skin. I focused so intently on my actions that I began to forget about my feelings. When I thought about them, I noticed they weren't as potent anymore. They were turning. I came to think of myself as a slow cooker. I had to throw a lot of things into it and then wait a very long time. If I looked inside mid-cook, it might not appear as though anything was happening. It would have been frustrating to peek into the pot too often, which is why it was important not to evaluate myself based on how I felt on any one day. I was an accumulation of all my days, good and bad. I can never know for sure what the single most helpful thing was for me, because in the end everything blended into one stew. I just know that it worked, and in time I became well again.

* * *

Luckily, as far as the outside world was concerned, Jeremy and I managed to keep our careers afloat. Jeremy was doing a good job managing *Tracktown*'s distribution and generally maintaining our professional relationships in the film world. And as I felt more stable and healthy internally, I was able to direct my gaze outward and begin piecing together how I'd move forward. This was a much healthier approach than what I had taken before, which was to attempt to solve my inner despair by desperately trying to control the outside world. I thought that external things, like shoe contracts and injuries, were what caused my depression and by fixing those I could fix myself. But what I learned was that it was important to solve my internal problems with *internal* solutions before I could reengage with the external world.

My first move was to see if I could undo the contract I signed with Nike in the darkest moment of my crisis. Dr. Arpaia helped me understand that I hadn't been thinking with rational perspective, and I knew now that a small Nike contract would not be in my best interest, especially since I really did want to move to Mammoth Lakes and train at altitude full-time. It would be better to be an unpaid free agent in Mammoth Lakes than an underpaid Nike athlete for the four-year duration of the contract I had signed. Dr. Arpaia encouraged me to be honest with Nike about what I had been going through when I signed the agreement.

Admitting to Nike that I had had a mental crisis was very hard for me. I was nervous about what they would say. I was afraid they would laugh at me, or not take me seriously, or think I was incompetent or even a bad person. When I finally had the courage to admit what was going on and ask that my contract be canceled, none of my fears came true. The team at Nike appreciated my honesty and they compassionately released me from the contract. Even though we were now officially without our main source of income, I felt light as Jeremy and I loaded up a U-Haul and drove back to Mammoth Lakes with all our belongings, ready to make our new start, for real this time.

I took some time without a contract so that I could regain my footing and figure out what was most important to me. I knew what I ideally wanted out of a partnership: a company that embraced me for exactly what I was, an athlete *and* an artist. I worked up the courage to reach out to Champion, a brand I'd long admired, and although they had never sponsored a professional runner before, we were such a good fit that they put together an apparel deal for me on an unprecedented basis. It was a dream come true that I never could have imagined during my depression. They valued my athletics, my film work, and my well-rounded persona. They celebrated and amplified my voice. Most importantly, I believed in their clothing and I knew that I would be honored to wear a Champion uniform on a starting line.

* * *

Conquering my depression was the hardest and bravest thing I've ever done. I can't emphasize that enough. During my depression, I felt embarrassed about it. I told my dad that I was sure I would feel depressed forever and that it would be embarrassing to continue living this way, so maybe it was better to just die. But then my dad said that being dead would be more embarrassing than being depressed. I really appreciated his thoughtful doses of humor and reality. Now I feel proud because I am still alive. Honestly, that's how bad it got.

Throughout the ordeal, my dad kept telling me I would get

something out of this that I'd never had before. I kept telling him I *had it all* before and that I didn't believe I could be happier than I had been—but the truth was, I didn't have it all. Before my depression, I always knew that the trajectory of my career was entirely in my own hands, but what I didn't understand is that my emotions could also be in my control. I used to think that my feelings were not up to me, that they were uncontrollable reactions to the world around me and all I could do was hope for more good feelings than bad ones. But now I know better.

I also used to think my depression was a test from my mom, or a punishment. When my mom killed herself, it planted a little seed of fear that one day I'd end up like her. That seed took root and became a part of me—as Dr. Arpaia described it, it became a "personal law." And when we have personal laws that are powerful enough, we tend to let our life play out in scenarios echoing that specific personal law. Me, I was most afraid of becoming so sad that I'd want to quit and leave this life. And it nearly happened—subconsciously, our minds want to prove our personal laws true.

All of us carry personal laws into our daily lives, usually without any clue as to what they actually are, and as a result we find ourselves thinking or feeling or behaving irrationally in certain situations without knowing why. The simplest way to understand personal laws is to think of them like food poisoning for your brain.

Once I got very sick after eating ratatouille infused with saffron, and now, years later, the smell of saffron is a trigger that causes my stomach to shut down. Even if it's something as safe and simple as a side of saffron white rice, my body will irrationally reject it. My brain created a personal law: Saffron is bad. Dr. Arpaia explained that the brain's purpose is self-preservation—but the problem is, the brain goes into overdrive and starts recognizing the personal law in places it shouldn't. Even though I know that plain bowl of saffron white rice is perfectly safe, it makes me sick anyway.

The brain behaves similarly with emotional trauma: When we create a personal law in response to trauma, the law can become hardwired into your brain so strongly that when you encounter even vaguely similar situations much later, your mind reacts with irrational intensity. I had a personal law that I had the same weakness as my mom, and I was interpreting my post-Olympic depression as proof that I was turning out like her.

In reflecting on my life even before my depression, I can see how I had unconsciously replicated some of the most painful experiences my mother impressed upon me. It affected other things beyond the depressive thoughts, such as my mindset that I deserved certain things because of my tough experience with my mother, or that I couldn't trust people, or that I could and should just cut people out of my life as she did to me. I didn't want to be vulnerable to the loneliness that she left for me, but in trying to avoid loneliness, I became even lonelier. I had been using my negative personal law about my mom as a protective mechanism for myself, which is as potent as it is unsustainable. Leaning on this personal law made me feel so deserving that I unrelentingly pushed until I got to the Olympics, but it also created uglier behaviors that left me very isolated, desperate, and at times, a very bad friend to people I loved. By trying to not be my mother, I became more like her. No matter how much I had accomplished on the outside, inside, I had a long way to go. I was living my life, but I was also missing out on my life because I had personal laws I did not fully understand.

I worked hard. This was not about developing my body, as I was so accustomed to, this was about evolving my mind. With help from Dr. Arpaia, I managed to break free of my negative personal law about my mom and emerge safely on the other side. He helped me understand that although my personal laws might *feel* real, they are not real. Who I am is still forever affected by my mom's actions, but now I understand that I can either be hostage to my past or accept it as some kind of beginning to what I will become. If a bad thing happens, you can see it as a harbinger of more bad things to come or as an opportunity for growth. Both mindsets represent ways to survive in the world, but one makes you a victim while the other empowers you. It's easier to be a victim; it takes bravery to claim your power.

My mother wasn't trying to hurt me from afar; she is dead. The only muscles a dead person has are the ones we invent for them. I am not my mother and she was not herself and I never knew her but I am made of her—I always wanted to know her, but now I know that the best way to get to know her is to get to know myself. These days I think of her like Puck from *A Midsummer Night's Dream*: She's mischievous but fundamentally good-hearted. When I have good luck I like to credit her, and when I have bad luck I like to think it's because she's lovingly keeping me grounded. But my mother is not in control—it is my responsibility and also my privilege to lead the life I want, despite my past (and regardless of whatever trickery Puck throws my way).

In fact, I can make *new* personal laws that make my life better. Every night I spend time cultivating my positive personal laws, like a farmer: The world is rooting for me, I am deserving, I am safe. Our personal laws can be our greatest crutch or our greatest asset. They also don't need to be things that just happen to us; they are things we can actually create for ourselves.

That's what being a Bravey is—you are making a conscious choice to tell yourself what you'd like to be until it becomes part of you. You choose to replace "can't" with "maybe" by acknowledging your feelings but focusing on your actions. Your actions encompass everything from what you do with your time, to who you surround yourself with, to the words you feed your mind. To know you can do this for yourself is the most powerful thing in the world.

Now, on the other side of the darkest time in my life, I understand what my dad meant when he said that I could conquer this and end up better than before. Even though it nearly killed me, I achieved what my mom could not.

Braveys, just know that however sad or depressed you might feel, I promise that I have felt the worst of it, too. And you *can* get better. It's a fact. It doesn't happen all at once—it starts with sporadic moments of hope in a sea of gloom, then there will be whole days where you don't have one bad thought, and then eventually your good days will outnumber your bad days and you'll realize that you are happy. I know from experience. It was the hardest thing I ever did. I don't have regrets, I have tools. I am so happy that I did it. I am so happy.

When I felt my happiness return, I knew that I would never again be afraid to fail. I felt like I was flying. For the first time in my life, I was fearless.

girl: u ever get sad

wildflower: why

girl: u only bloom for a few weeks out of the year

wildflower: doesn't make me sad

girl: how come

wildflower: all the other weeks matter too

girl: how

wildflower: i'm resting, preparing, growing, becoming . . .

girl: oh!

wildflower: i'm here all year even if u can't see me

girl: forever wildflower

JERRY SEINFELD

Jerry Seinfeld's voice echoed through my childhood home like I imagined a mother's might. Whether it was breakfast or dinnertime, Jerry would be jabbering at whoever happened to be passing by the TV in the living room, or sometimes to no audience at all. Jerry's musings about where the caffeine goes in decaf coffee or why you park on a driveway but drive on a parkway were like the sounds of traffic outside a big-city apartment, constant and soothing. We didn't like a quiet house and Jerry always had something to say.

Jerry liked to talk about minutiae, which was perfect. No subject was too small to catapult him into a monologue about his amusement, dissatisfaction, annoyance, or pleasure. I loved getting lost in his obsession over the little things: jackets, Chinese restaurants, nonfat yogurt, Junior Mints. I took comfort in Jerry's world where everything was worthy of discussion, letting his thoughts and opinions steep in my mind like tea leaves in hot water. It was distracting in a good way; in my house, we did not want to talk about the big stuff, the messy stuff. I knew certain topics were off-limits with my dad and brother. But anything was fair game with Jerry. His voice filled the silence.

We hardly ever talked about our feelings in my family. Instead, we took action: If you are tired, you sleep. If you are sad, you cry. If you are angry, you throw a temper tantrum or, in my brother's case, you beat up your little sister. But talking about the sad feelings that made you cry or the mad feelings that made you lose control, that was just *not done*. If I was upset, I cried until all the rage was gone while my dad said, "I know, I know, I'm sorry," as if these feelings were just waves that I needed to ride out. Trying to reason with my feelings would be as useless as a sailor trying to negotiate with the waves. Better to ride them out when they come. Maybe my dad felt that it was too hard to engage with the emotions that take hold of two young kids whose mom has died by suicide. Suicide isn't something people like to talk about but that doesn't mean the feelings are going to disappear. They'll just come out in a different way, like tipping a bookshelf onto your sister or screaming at the top of your lungs until you lose your voice and you can't anymore.

I didn't find out how my mom really died until I was in seventh grade, when we were supposed to write tombstones for people we knew who had died from smoking. You see, before that, I thought my mom died from smoking because I knew she smoked and in school we learned that *smoking kills*. I dedicated my cardboard tombstone to my mother. My mother's *Roberta Pappas* tombstone was surrounded by a sea of *Walt Disney*s, because someone whispered that he had died from lung cancer and so everyone else wrote his name. I felt brave for writing my mom's name, as if I was honoring her and, in this way, expressing my love for her.

But then on the bus ride home that day, my best friend, Amanda, told me that her mom told her that my mom had killed herself. Everybody knew but me. Amanda cried when she shared this news with me. But I didn't cry. I used to feel sorry for my mom, because I thought she was just ignorant to the negative consequences of smoking. I saw her as a victim. I felt like she was by my side. But then a little stew of rage welled up inside of me: She left. Fuck her, I thought. She's *out*.

* * *

Every Mother's Day, my dad would take my brother and me to visit our mom's grave so we could take turns talking to her tombstone. When it was my turn I would tell her about my day, how I was doing in school, and how I missed her and hoped she was well. I always asked her to please keep my dad, brother, cat, and friends happy, healthy, and alive. But after I learned how she actually died, I refused to visit her grave for the next five years. I would have rather talked to a regular stone than to hers.

I never felt angry with my dad or brother for not telling me sooner how she really died. All my anger was reserved for my mom. I felt like I knew her even less than I thought I did.

I was insatiably curious but I never tried to pry for more information about her from my dad or brother. I didn't want to hurt them by stirring up something that we had come to accept was beyond the reach of words. The result is that I basically knew nothing about her. There were no stories or anecdotes, just a few facts: She went to Goucher College, she went to Hebrew school with Ben of Ben & Jerry's, she liked to sing, and she was athletic. Facts can be important, but they're hard to visualize on their own. I wanted *stories* so I could understand where I came from. I worried constantly—how could I make sure not to end up like her if I had no idea who she was in the first place? I didn't want to be mad at her anymore; being mad is exhausting. Now I wanted to *understand* her.

In college I took a class called Women and Madness, an intersectional course between the Psychology and the Women's Studies departments, to see if I could understand my mother better. The class focused on the cultural evolution of mental illness in women, specifically how our culture has handled its diagnosis and treatment from one generation to the next. I learned that during the late 1980s, when women in my mom's generation were fully entering the corporate world alongside men, there was tremendous social pressure not to complain about anything that bothered them, big or small. They were told to be grateful for their newly upgraded status in society, and that complaining about the pressures of balancing a career with all the expectations of motherhood was seen as weakness or even proof that the women's rights movement was wrong. I knew vaguely that my mother had some sort of computer-related corporate career; could she have been caught up in the societal pressure that I was learning about?

I called my dad to get more information. "What did Mommy do for her job before she got sick?" I asked him. (My dad, my brother, and I have maintained the habit of calling her "Mommy" throughout the years, as if to suspend her in time; she was a *Mommy* when she died and she will stay that way forever.) He told me that my mom taught herself computer programming, becoming one of the first Kelly Girls (the name for women who worked for Kelly Services, a well-known temp agency) to earn a full-time position at the database management firm where she was assigned to work. But her promising career was cut short by a severe case of scoliosis, which led to an addiction to painkillers, drug abuse, and being diagnosed as bipolar with manic depression. She actually stole her doctors' prescription pads, forged prescriptions for Vicodin, and strategically redeemed them at boutique pharmacies throughout the East Bay where there wasn't a computer system that could track her purchases from one location to the next. My dad didn't figure it out until it was too late—like I said, she was very smart and capable. In fact, she was abusing painkillers throughout her pregnancy with me, which is probably why I get sick whenever I need to take painkillers today. The pieces fit: In my mind, I crafted a narrative for my mother as a groundbreaker on the cutting edge of women in the workplace, but who cracked under the pressure of juggling her career, motherhood, and a medical disability.

But the more facts I learned about my mother, the more it was clear that I really didn't know *her* at all. So finally, in May 2018, one month before I got married, I asked my dad to give me just one thing as a wedding gift: stories about my mother. I made the ask when I was visiting for a wedding-dress fitting, and I wasn't sure how he would take my request. He told me he'd see what he could do, and we left it at that; neither of us brought it up again for the rest of the visit. Then, moments before I had to leave for the airport, he handed me a folded-up packet of paper.

It was my mom's eulogy, written by the rabbi who performed her funeral service. It had been written on a typewriter and felt to me like a stage prop. As I unfolded the creased yellow pages, I felt like I was watching myself in a movie—the scene where the character finds a long-lost artifact about her mysterious past, or maybe a treasure map. But the words on those pages were very real. It hurt me to even hold them because I knew it would hurt me to read them. As I hugged my dad goodbye, I felt a tremendous tenderness toward him. He had made himself vulnerable by handing me this packet of paper, a document that he had clearly kept safely hidden for decades because he was too upset or afraid or unprepared to share its existence with me before. I read it on the flight and I cried the whole time. There was one passage in particular that meant so much to me:

> Robbie could never be still. She had boundless energy and endurance. She sang in the temple choir and the San Francisco Symphony choir. She would come back from a hike and go bicycling. She would get off the airplane in New York to visit her brother and immediately go jogging. Nevermind it was dark and she didn't know the neighborhood and there were no streetlights. There was no deterring Robbie . . . she brought her knitting when she went sailing. But for all her extroversion, for all her overwhelming friendliness, her welcoming of strangers into her house, her fearlessness in tackling the world, Robbie rarely let her friends scratch the surface. She maintained that things were always wonderful, and, even when others knew they weren't, she protected herself so valiantly from letting them see deep inside. Robbie was alone with her torment.

There it was. Just one paragraph was all it took for me to completely understand my mother—because she reminded me exactly of myself. Like her, I never stop moving or trying or pushing or doing. She and I are similar in so many ways, ways I cannot possibly change. But there is one stark difference: Unlike my mother, I choose to let people in. I choose to share what is going on in my mind so that I'm never alone with my torment. I conquered my post-Olympic depression because I shared my feelings with my dad and then, finally, with a really good doctor. I was not alone with my torment, and I know that is why I'm still here today, writing this book.

My mom felt ashamed of her struggles and tried to keep everything hidden. She didn't want people to know how she felt. But now everyone's going to know. I'm going to tell them because everyone can learn from this. It's too big for me to hold all alone. Death is private but suicide belongs to everyone.

* * *

What's funny is that after I finished reading my mom's eulogy, I thought about Jerry Seinfeld. I finally understood why his "show about nothing" amounted to something quite significant. Because when you *don't* talk about something, it becomes like hair in a shower drain: invisible for a while but building up over time into a slimy, obtrusive clump.

My mother's whole emotional existence occurred inside of herself, whereas Jerry lets his feelings out like dandelion seeds on the wind. By musing on things that seem small, he gives us permission to consider *anything* worthy of discussion. Everybody hates some things, and everybody experiences pain. Everybody has a hard day or days, or days and days. But in Jerry's world, no single thing can become big enough to destroy us. We might even find humor in the things that bother us most.

From now until forever, *someone* will know everything about me. It doesn't need to be the same person, and it certainly doesn't need to be everybody—but whether I've had a bad turkey sandwich or dropped out of a workout or experienced something even more painful, somebody will know it and they will help hold that thing with me.

I wish I could have taught my mom what Jerry taught me: to just let it out and be unselfconsciously honest. The only way to not be *forever sad* is to admit that we are, for the moment, *sad*. I have heard that comedians are some of the saddest people on earth, and I have no idea if that's true, but maybe that's why I love them. Inside of me is my mother, who was one of the saddest people on earth. Sadness was my inheritance. And while I know sharing everything isn't a foolproof method, it has proven very useful to me. Everything inside of me is also somewhere outside of me. I don't want to stay behind with them, the things inside. I want to make room for the next thing life hands me and the next and the next, because I expect there will *always* be a next.

When I finally had the chance to see Jerry Seinfeld perform stand-up live, it made me cry. The whole auditorium was laughing, but I was crying. I was so touched to see him in person. The dependable friend who ate dinner with us every night during my childhood finally had a real body and a heartbeat. Even though I was just one member of a huge audience in a big theater, in that moment I felt like I was home.

i know you watch me sleep

view how i turn in the night

see how i dress in the morn

feel when i turn out my light

hear me make a great yell

with someone out of your sight

goldfish i've never touched you

but i want to hug you so tight.

WILLPOWER

It's impossible to tell how sad or happy or out of their mind someone is by looking at their handwriting. Handwriting can be calm even when you are a storm. When I was rummaging through my dad's garage over a holiday trip home, I found a box containing medical records from my mother's institutionalization. The box was buried deep behind an old rowboat that must not have been touched in over fifteen years. In the box, among pages of dusty medical reports, were a few precious pieces of paper in my mom's handwriting from her mental-ward days and, really, you wouldn't be able to tell from her perfect cursive that she was right on the edge.

The pages with her handwriting were worksheets of self-help exercises that the hospital staff made her fill out. They were mostly focused on trying to change the way she felt about herself.

The hospital kept my mom very busy with these assignments, all of which looked like they were designed for a first-grader, complete with little pictures and text in juvenile fonts. One of the worksheets was titled "Who Am I?" in Comic Sans font, with fill-in-the-blank lines where my mom wrote all the things she *was*: mother, daughter, student, homeowner, wife, patient, disciplinarian, singer, musician. Then there was another set of blank lines for her to put things she does well and things "to be improved" for each of these roles.

She filled in the blanks with nice, controlled handwriting and carefully composed sentences. In the "to be improved" space, she wrote banal suggestions to incorporate into her mothering routine: "Limits & consequences. i.e: timeout for not listening. Setting limits. First timeout, then no TV, then no soccer class." She also wrote, "I am angry with myself for not keeping my professional technical skills current and for letting other people raise my kids for me."

Her perfect cursive is what kills me. This is coming from a woman who had just been readmitted to the psychiatric ward for heavy drug abuse and who would later try to saw her own arm off in her bathroom. Yet according to these fill-in-the-blank mental-health worksheets, her top priorities were to keep her work skills current and whether timeout should come before no TV. Fuck, Mom. I mean, *fuck*. It's clear that she cared very much about being a mother, which makes me very sad.

Of all the mental hospital worksheets I found, the alphabet one stings me the most. It's called "I Like Myself A to Z!" Except my mom inserted *WILL!* between *I* and *Like* so that the revised title of the worksheet was "I WILL! Like Myself A to Z!" Beneath the title, the alphabet was spelled out in an infantile font with a blank space after each letter for her to fill in an adjective about herself. The answers were all in her handwriting, but I noticed some of them were crossed out and rewritten, probably with guidance from a therapist. She originally wrote things like *T* is for *tiny* but then it was crossed out and replaced with *tenacious*. *O* was originally for *overcommitted* but then she crossed it out and wrote *overcomer*. *N* was *narcissistic*, revised to *likes to nurse others*. *Self-centered* became *serious*. I assume the replacement was meant to be the better thing, the thing she was trying to force herself to become.

But what's so bad about a mentally ill person being *self-centered*? Being mentally ill is the perfect time to be self-centered. At least that was my experience. When I was severely depressed, focusing exclusively on myself and my healing was the only way I was able to save my own life. I understand very well that when you are depressed, your mind is injured. You cannot understand yourself and your place in the world. It frustrates me that my mom did not have good help; it frustrates me that she was trying to be there for other people before she was able to be there for herself.

What makes me sad and also angry is that these hospital-administered worksheets reinforced labels that my mom should have let go of for the sake of her own health: Homeowner, computer programmer, wife, mother. The mental healthcare system responsible for my mom's rehabilitation valued preserving these labels over maintaining the person underneath them, as if they could wrap her up with enough "wife" and "mother" and "computer programmer" bandages to repair the hurt she felt inside, or at least to keep her depression as invisible as possible. But all they did was turn her into a mummy. Her labels suffocated her until she couldn't take it anymore. She needed to treat her internal problems, as I did when I was depressed, before thinking about her external responsibilities. Although she was mentally ill, my mother did not have to die—depression is not a terminal illness—it was the healthcare system at that time, with its unyielding attachment to socially acceptable labels, that killed her. My mother wasn't alone: In the course of doing research for this book, my dad shared the staggering fact that of my mother's six closest girlfriends during her young professional years in the Bay Area, *three* of them died by suicide. (One of the women who died was my mom's maid of honor.)

People should be allowed breaks from their labels, especially if it is to save their own life. If a person is not answering to their number one task, to take care of themselves, then they shouldn't have to take on any other responsibilities. You have to take care of yourself first. You are your own most precious resource. Everything you are in this world hinges on you facing yourself before you face the world. The problem with those worksheets is that they never allowed my mom to disengage from her responsibilities, even for a little while, for the sake of the *self*—the person, naked, without any labels but her name: Roberta.

* * *

Looking at my life from the outside, it's clear that I do many things at once: I run, I write, I act, and I even make homemade sourdough bread. But what isn't as obvious is all the things I'm *not* doing. For example, even if you can't tell from my social media feed, I rarely do much creative work on the days I have hard workouts. I can do many things, but not all at once— I know and respect that on workout days, my body and mind are tired and just need to rest. I am kind to myself in this way.

I wasn't always kind to myself, though. I used to think that I always needed to be pushing myself harder, further, grinding more . . . and, like my mom, I'd get frustrated and upset if I felt like I was underperforming in any situation, no matter what extenuating circumstances there might have been. I had a bizarre internal struggle with the reality that I had resources in my life that my mom simply did not have. At its best, it made me feel grateful. At its worst, it made me feel spoiled. I felt a mountain of pressure on myself to succeed, because unlike my mom, I had everything I needed, so I'd better do it right. I did not understand that I could be kind to myself and still want more out of myself at the same time.

In college, we were assigned a book to read called *Willpower* by Roy Baumeister and John Tierney. Their thesis states that our ability to make constructive choices and accomplish things is governed by our willpower, and our willpower for a given day is finite. When our willpower is depleted we are less likely to be disciplined about the choices we make and less likely to be effective in whatever we're trying to do. Willpower is a *measurable* and *depletable* resource.

We make thousands of choices every day, and each of those choices uses up some portion of our willpower. The little decisions—when to wake up, what to eat, what to wear, when to leave the house—are small paper cuts that deplete the willpower that *could have* gone toward bigger decisions: Should I study for that test or watch TV? Can I finish this workout or should I give up? We need to be conscious of what decisions we're allowing to use up our limited supply of willpower. Once I started becoming conscious of my own willpower, and then protective of it, two things began to happen: I became kinder to myself when my willpower was low, and I realized how many little things drained my willpower every day.

When I went to my first altitude training camp as a pro runner, I came up with a concept called "willpower budgeting," which means proactively shaping the day ahead to make sure my willpower goes where it needs to go. This was an invention of necessity because at high altitude, everything is harder on your body. Since there's less oxygen, your body works significantly harder to run paces that would be easy at sea level *and* your body requires much more recovery than normal. At altitude camp I felt like I was hitting a wall every day. I wanted to do more with my time than I felt physically capable of doing. So I decided to evaluate my willpower situation. Were there areas where I could "save" willpower? In other words, I made a willpower budget.

When making a willpower budget, the best place to start is with the little things: How can you cut out some of the smaller day-to-day decisions that use up little drops of willpower? For me, having a set routine for the day ahead is key. I coined one of my favorite personal mantras, "Tomorrow Starts Tonight," because before I go to bed I lay out my clothes, pack my day bag, set up my coffee pot, and even write a to-do list and schedule. Every micro-decision that I can make for myself ahead of time leaves me more willpower to dedicate to training the next morning, or to whatever big task is on my plate. If you're planning your day on the fly, there's no way it'll be as efficient. I also started becoming more vigilant with medium and big decisions: I was much more thoughtful about how much I committed to in a single day, and I made sure that all of my tasks had a set starting time and place. I was no longer down to "meet at 3-ish for a run somewhere," because I understood that the back-and-forth texting leading up to the run would cost me some willpower. It's much easier to take the time to make thoughtful plans. On any given day, I'm never quite sure if I'll even be able to physically do what my coach wants me to do. But every morning, I *do* know where to be and when. And so on hard training days, from the moment I wake up until the moment I start my first rep, all I need to think about is the workout.

Before I was aware of willpower budgeting, I used to find myself getting upset and feeling bitter in situations that were willpower draining. On team van rides to workouts I'd be chatting with my teammates for the entire forty-five-minute drive down the mountain, but inside I'd feel drained. I am an introvert, so while I love conversation and social interactions, I am not energized by them. I require lots of alone time. But once I started thinking more proactively about my willpower, I started bringing along headphones so that when I needed to, I could remove myself from the team chitchat and just stay focused on the task. At first I felt selfish doing this, like I should entertain all the conversations happening around me, but now I understand that in order to contribute the most to the world, I need to be protective of my willpower.

* * *

The best way to budget your willpower is to know yourself and understand what drains your willpower and what replenishes it. Jeremy and I developed a visual tool to help us understand this, the Willpower Index.

The idea for the index came about when I was recovering from an injury and had to exercise on an indoor stationary bike every day. Even though I knew that some people would *love* to spend two hours each morning biking alone in a gym, I hated it. I wanted to be running outside with my team, not stuck indoors on the bike. Then I would get mad at myself for not appreciating that I "get to bike" while other people who might love biking can't because of their full-time jobs. It was a negative feedback loop: I was upset that I had to bike, then I'd get *more* upset that I was upset.

But that's not how willpower works. Willpower is different for everyone, and I was comparing my personal willpower standards to an objective standard for what I thought I *should* feel. That's where the index comes in.

The Willpower Index is a simple table with an X and a Y axis. The Y axis represents a range from "bad for you" to "good for you." The X axis represents "willpower draining" to "willpower boosting."

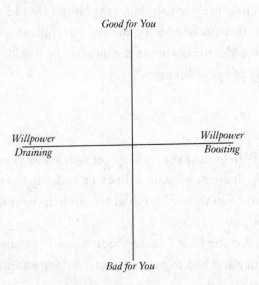

For me, biking is "good for me" but "willpower draining," whereas for someone else, biking might be "good for me" and "willpower boosting." I understand I am biking for a good reason, but it is still draining my willpower. A night of partying might be "bad for me" but "willpower boosting," and a night spent on a red-eye flight is "bad for me" and "willpower draining." And so on.

The point is, as you budget your willpower, it's helpful to evaluate what activities are actually willpower boosting versus draining to you personally, and also to make sure that there aren't too many hours in your day clustered in one particular area of the chart. In the team van on the way to practice, chitchat with my teammates is willpower draining—but for someone else, it could just as easily be willpower boosting. I try not to judge myself when I look at how my day spreads out along this chart, but I do pay attention to a balance. If my day is filled with "willpower draining" activities, then it makes sense that I feel exhausted. You wouldn't get frustrated with yourself for feeling hungry if you haven't eaten, so why get frustrated if you need to boost your willpower when it's low?

When I started understanding my willpower in this way, not only did I have more energy to accomplish more things but, most important, I stopped beating myself up when I *didn't* have energy. That's the beauty of understanding willpower: We become kinder to ourselves.

I love cooking, but I always used to rush through it because I saw cooking as a nonproductive use of time, something to be completed as quickly as possible. But now that I understand cooking is a "willpower boosting" activity for me, I allow myself to lean in and enjoy it. I feel deserving of it. Likewise, I listen to podcasts on long drives. They're "good for me" and "willpower boosting." I like to listen to podcasts of interviews with people I admire. On a recent drive from Oregon to California, I listened to an interview with Natalie Portman where she talks about how she balances everything: acting, motherhood, and daily life. She explains that for her the key is accepting that she isn't going to be perfect. She says: "I always have avocado on my shirt or I've gone into so many meetings with my shirt unbuttoned because I've just been breastfeeding right before a meeting. I'm tired. I mess things up all the time because I'm so tired. I say things wrong, I make mistakes, I'm falling on my face, I'm not with my kids enough, I'm not doing my job well enough, like, as completely as I could, but I'm kind of comfortable with that. And I think that's kind of the secret for me, is like, you know, I'm trying my best and I forgive myself."

Natalie's words speak volumes about the concept of willpower. She recognizes that she only has so much energy, and by accepting that fact, she is okay and even thriving within such a hectic life. That's what willpower is all about. Natalie says she knows herself and feels comfortable with herself, and that the secret to being a good mom (or a good anything) is to be okay trying *your* best.

In my own life, every day is a balancing act between my athletic training and any number of creative projects, business emails, and conference calls. Some days I feel like Superwoman and other days I simply have to let certain things go. From time to time, I need to be okay being *good enough*. Natalie is a role model for me because she is someone who is as kind to herself as she is hard on herself. She understands that her willpower is finite and she is okay with that. I wish my mom could have met

Natalie, or what I really mean is, I wish I could meet Natalie and I wish my mom could have met me.

Being as kind to yourself as you are hard on yourself is a skill that I've had to actively nurture. I had a teammate at UO named Becca who, when she felt particularly overwhelmed or otherwise dissatisfied with her day, would put on PJs, get into bed, turn off the lights, lie down for one minute, and then spring out of bed and declare "NEW DAY!," put on a new outfit, make coffee, and have breakfast again. It didn't matter if it was ten in the morning or six at night—if she sensed her day going south, she allowed herself this routine. It is the ultimate self-kindness.

* * *

At my dad's second wedding, which happened shortly before I turned twenty-nine, the guest list was just shy of three hundred people. Everyone I've known since I was four years old was there, along with my entire new extended family of dozens of step-aunts, -uncles, and -cousins. Kristina, my new stepmom, grew up in the Bay Area and her expansive Chinese-American family is very close-knit. There are contingents of her family that are still in Hong Kong and Canton, but the Chinese-American side has been here for generations. I've never been part of a big family, and I was grateful that my extended family was more than quadrupling in size. Kristina pulled me aside and told me that if and when I have a baby she would be by my side and make me traditional Chinese black vinegar ginger pig's-feet stew to help with postnatal healing. This maternal gesture from Kristina made me feel cared for and included in our new family. Among the few guests from my dad's side was one of my mom's best friends, Abbe. Abbe has always taken the time to tell me how great my dad is and also how proud my mom would have been of how we all turned out.

On this particular night, in the middle of the Chinese dragon dance, I found myself at Abbe's table. She told me, as she always does, how proud she was of me and how my mom would have also been tremendously proud. This always gets to me in a place I can't pinpoint, somewhere under my ribs, which, if it were poked too hard, would make me literally fall over. I don't know how I feel about hearing that my mom would have been proud of me.

I associate the emotion of parental pride with a sense of feeling like you are, in fact, a good parent. You are proud of your kid but you are also proud of yourself. I feel sad that my mom can't be here to feel proud, since, according to Abbe, she wanted desperately to be a good mom. And so I feel sad in these moments that my mom will never be able to feel the pride she surely would have felt if she had stayed alive. It's probably why I am an overachiever—because I will prove to her and to myself that, yeah, she missed out on a lot.

As the dragon dancers jumped on each other's shoulders, beating their drums louder, Abbe told me how my mom worked very hard to be there for us, how she took us to tumbling and then to the park and then taught us extra lessons at home from *Early World of Learning* encyclopedia books. In fact, my mom sold these children's encyclopedias door-to-door in our neighborhood to other young moms as a side business during the period of time when she was unable to work due to her medical disabilities. It was not big money, but it was something she enjoyed doing: going to peoples' houses and giving sales-pitch presentations. I imagine she also craved the sense of purpose she felt as a saleswoman, which makes me proud and also very sad.

She tried so hard. But no matter how hard my mom tried, she didn't end up turning out okay. And then I get even sadder because, well, somehow my brother and I turned out okay without her and even *despite* her, so she might as well have worried about herself and not us. Instead of using those silly hospital worksheets to agonize over how to be a better mother, maybe if she had channeled all her energy into *herself* and forgotten about us kids for a while, she would have been able to be there for herself and then, eventually, for us. Maybe if she had taken one or two years off of mothering and her career to focus on healing, she might have had thirty or forty or fifty more years to experience being a mother and businesswoman.

Looking at it now, it's an obvious trade. But I'm sure that for my mom things weren't as clear. Every day that she spent in the hospital must have been doubly painful for her because not only was she unwell but she was also "neglecting" my brother and me. She thought she had to manage it all at once but she couldn't, and life began to feel impossible. Trying to grapple with *impossible* is like trying to use tweezers to grab a cloud. You can't. And so the pressure built until she killed herself. Unlike me, my mom wasn't able to understand her own willpower.

And while most people aren't in as desperate a situation as my mom was, many of us still have trouble seeing the forest for the trees when it comes to how we spend our willpower. We are so focused on what we think we *should be* doing that we make unwise choices about what is truly best for us.

* * *

My mom's maiden name was North and I think it's funny she
lives in the sky.

After I read through her handwritten worksheets, I took the
time to read every page of her medical reports from the mental
ward. I used to wonder if I made it all up; the horrible things I
saw could not be real. But there they were, in ink on paper. The
documents confirmed that my mom did in fact lacerate her arm
with a saw as I remember, that I found her and saved her life,
and that then, when they institutionalized her, she lit herself on
fire in her hospital bed.

Going from those stark reports, dry and clinical in their language, to reading her childlike worksheets was enough to break
my heart. I got so sad when I read in her little cursive writing:
"Know it's the behavior you don't like. I love the child, not the
behavior." I am sure my brother and I misbehaved. I was four
and he was eight and we were both confused. I am sure we misbehaved. But we were kids.

Did she think we were watching her? I think I both was and
wasn't, watching her but not judging her. I probably just wanted
to spend time with her, but I would have gladly waited. This is
a key thing to understand when you're feeling low on willpower: The world will be okay without you while you recharge,
and in the long run, it will be even *better*. Reading my mom's
medical records drove the point home: There's no escaping the
hard truth that each of us has a fixed amount of willpower, a
certain amount of ability to deal with the shit the world throws
at us, and no amount of trying and straining can give us more.
We are the most honest things, us humans. We are squishy
pulses that see things, take them in, feel them inside, and regur-

gitate them in one way or another while we continue to roll around on this earth.

My mom must have thought that she could see forward in time, which is why she decided to kill herself. She was so overwhelmed that she assumed she'd never find a way out. When she thought about the future, she imagined descending further and further into doom. But nothing is forever. The only truth about the future is that we don't know what it is. Life can be better than you could ever imagine. It can be easy to forget this sometimes, especially when your willpower is low. In those moments, you can only see yourself through a mirror that is warped and distorted—and the mirror seems like it reflects on itself forever. It's impossible to try to look into the future this way because no matter how hard you try, you're still right there blocking your own view.

My mom only saw herself through the right-now mirror. If she had stopped straining to see the future beyond her right-now reflection and just made eye contact with herself, she would have seen that she was only human just like everyone else. Up close, you are exactly who you are right now. You might be sad or happy or chasing a dream or still trying to find one, but whatever you are, you are the truth. Right now, you are perfect.

you can be proud of yourself

and want more out of yourself

at the same time

BOYS VS. GIRLS

I grew up in a house of boys. My small T-shirts would get lost among the button-downs, undershirts, and dress socks that filled the washing machine. My brightly colored underwear, on the other hand, was always embarrassingly easy to find. The crisp freshness of men's deodorant and shaving cream wafted through our hallways, the scent as much of a morning staple as Eggo waffles in the toaster and Howard Stern blasting from my brother's radio. I felt comfortable in this masculine environment; it was normal to me.

Decor has never been my dad's strength. Other than my bedroom, which was a study in girlie overcompensation with a tiny pink chandelier and a *Beauty and the Beast* bedspread, our house was pretty empty except for four categories of items: baseball bobblehead collectible dolls, newspapers, clean unfolded laundry, and every trophy that my brother and I ever won. This was the 1990s, when people loved giant gaudy trophies. Every spare surface in the house was packed with trophies, with the occasional bobblehead (from the Giants' stadium, of course) wedged in. The floor, meanwhile, was covered in hundreds of newspapers. My dad began collecting newspapers around the time my mom died, and our house was essentially a newspaper maze with one narrow path carved through it. I was literally up to my waist in newspapers, hundreds and hundreds of them, dating back to 1995, the year my mom died. But really, if you removed just the newspapers and the laundry and the trophies and the bobbleheads, our house would have been quite empty.

Our refrigerator always had a gallon of two percent milk in it, and we never ran out of Diet Coke or food. My dad prepared dinner whenever he could, but it was also expected that you could handle feeding yourself if you were home alone and hungry. My dad insisted that we save all forms of plastic utensils and chopsticks from takeout orders, because we might need them, all 745 forks for the various meals we'd grab on the go between sporting events. The plasticware occupied one of the drawers in our kitchen island, and the other drawer overflowed with an endless pile of receipts and my dad's state quarter collection.

Essentially, our home was an overcrowded den where everything got lost and then found. Somehow everything got done. It was a bachelor pad if you considered both the dad and the kids as bachelors. There were no radio stations that were off-limits. When my brother and I were teenagers, there were some nights when all of us, including my dad, would be preparing to go out on dates at the same time. We would help each other pick outfits and then we'd fight over who got to use the car, as my perfume, my dad's aftershave, and my brother's cologne all mingled together.

There was no bedtime. We had a cat named Chloe (despite being a boy cat) and he was allowed to sleep anywhere he wanted and do whatever he wanted, just like the rest of us. In fact there were no household rules at all, except perhaps for the short

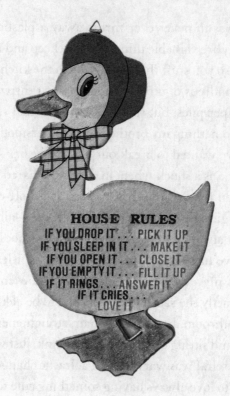

HOUSE RULES
IF YOU DROP IT . . . PICK IT UP
IF YOU SLEEP IN IT . . . MAKE IT
IF YOU OPEN IT . . . CLOSE IT
IF YOU EMPTY IT . . . FILL IT UP
IF IT RINGS . . . ANSWER IT
IF IT CRIES . . .
LOVE IT

phrases inscribed on the little wooden Mother Goose that hung above our landline phone.

The Mother Goose, along with a gigantic poster of the Giants' stadium displayed prominently as the focal point of the living room, where a family portrait might typically hang, were the only wall decorations we ever had in our house growing up. The Mother Goose was one of my mom's impulse purchases, but inexplicably the Mother Goose remained when all of her other belongings were removed from our home. I like to believe that Mother Goose's wide eye was an expression of approval and happiness rather than of shock and dismay at our unconventional household. In truth, the only household rule we *really* had to follow was to never ever throw away a plastic grocery bag because they are valuable things that we keep and never want to run out of, so you stuff them underneath the kitchen sink along with the hundreds of others. You also don't throw away any of the newspaper piles, but that was not an actual spoken rule, it was more something my brother and I understood we shouldn't do unless we wanted to break our daddy's heart.

So it came as a shock when, in college, I shared a living space with women for the first time. I lived in an off-campus house with other girls from the cross-country team—nine to be exact. There was always a mountain of running shoes by the front door and we had one bathroom between us. I learned how to distinguish my deodorant from the others even though they were all exactly the same, and I learned to be alert when entering the bathroom because the hair straightener was always turned on and sitting on the edge of the sink, just waiting for me to burn myself. I was wary of such a drastic change at first, but I soon came to love always having something cute to wear among nine shared wardrobes.

There was only one thing I had trouble adjusting to: the new rules of communication. In my childhood home, when you wanted something or had something to say about someone else in the household, you straight-up said it. If I was mad at my dad or brother, I said so and we fought. If my brother or I needed anything, we asked. We knew we had to advocate for ourselves. I sometimes pictured my friends' parents as owls, perched just above and hypervigilant for even the slightest sign that they needed to swoop in. That was not my dad. He simply needed to get through one day and then the next. My brother and I knew we needed to help him help us, and sometimes that meant speaking up.

But in my new house of girls, much was left unsaid. If after practice one of the girls said she was fine, it often meant she was actually *not fine*. If she said she was just okay, it meant *really-super-not-fine*. Like just-failed-an-exam not fine. Sometimes it was wise to ask what was wrong and to talk through problems with my teammates, but other times it was best to leave alone the things that felt beyond the reach of words. It was easy for me to fall into this new way of being; I *liked* being one of the girls, and lacking any other frame of reference, I figured that this silent communication method was just the way things were done. I became more demure and subtle. I hinted and suggested, never asserted or declared.

Then, sometime after I graduated, I found myself in a house with eight—eight!—boys when I was at altitude training camp in Flagstaff, Arizona. Not only was I the only girl in the house but I was the only girl in the entire training group at the time. Only one thing was the same as my time living with female teammates in college: the huge pile of running shoes by the front door. Everything else was different.

After our first hard workout at altitude, the boys and I were sitting around the kitchen eating eggs of various styles when one of them blurted out: "I felt like dog shit in that workout." Another boy burst through the bathroom door, towel around his waist, and announced that he'd had the best workout of his life and was *definitely* going to make the World Championship team that year. I looked up in surprise, expecting to find the other boys rolling their eyes, but all I saw was a chorus of nodding heads. I was totally taken aback at how casually these guys could express such dramatic and grandiose feelings, and how they all seemed to accept these proclamations at face value. The boys threw out big bold statements like confetti. Their descriptiveness was a creative triumph; their language was more vulgar, expressive, vivid, and creative than anything I ever heard my female teammates say in school. Such extreme proclamations felt characteristically *male* to me, like when my brother would tell me that I had BO or when my dad would tell me he needed to go to the bathroom *right now*. After my experience of living with girls, I had fallen out of practice with this direct way of communicating.

Then one of the boys turned to me: "How was the workout for you, Lex?"

I wasn't sure how to answer. I actually felt really great about my workout, but then I heard the words coming out of my mouth: "It was fine."

This broad application of the word *fine* to cover up any strong feelings seems distinctly female to me. I wonder if this was a phenomenon unique to my particular experience with my teammates at Dartmouth, or if it's a more universal trend among young women everywhere. I told myself to reconsider my choice of words, to open up and say how I really felt. No, the workout was not "fine," it had been *spectacular*. It was the best thing since sliced bread. I spoke again: "Actually, I fucking crushed today's workout." It felt extreme and dramatic to say it, but it also felt really good. It felt like confidence.

Eventually, though, I noticed a downside to this "masculine" form of self-expression. The very next day, the boy who said his workout was like dog shit let his proclamation hinder his training. He had declared the shittyness so strongly that he got inside his own head. Sure enough, I could see he was hypersensitive on the track—until he finally had a good workout the following day, so he could make a *new* proclamation that he was the best thing to happen to running since the invention of shoes. Yes, the boys made statements that seemed bold and confident, but their entire realities would shift with each new proclamation. They were on top of the world one day and then down in a gully the next. I started to see how making bold, declarative statements could become unproductive.

So which approach was better, the boys' or the girls'? Was it better to keep my feelings hidden under the blanket of *fine,* or to swing myself up and down like a yo-yo? I felt torn between extremes. I didn't care so much which behavior belonged to which gender; I just wanted to know what would help me be the best athlete.

This remained an unsolved question in my mind until one of my role models, Olympic silver medalist Sally Kipyego, taught me to think of my training as a series of boxes all of equal value. Each day, I tick a box. The hard-workout box is just as important as the recovery box, and it is crucial not to place too much emphasis on any single box, good or bad. What *is* crucial is to give a hundred percent of what you have every day, whether it's a hundred percent of crap or a hundred percent of gold. You acknowledge the day and move on to the next. You're not trying to ignore how you feel every day like my female teammates did when they said they were fine, nor are you constantly boomeranging between highs and lows like my male teammates. Instead, you're taking a more zoomed-out perspective of the journey. A training cycle should be seen as a long-term body of work, and any single day probably won't make or break your season.

The same principle applies to nonathletic pursuits as well, whether it's a creative project or a business career or even a relationship. Thinking about the pursuit of any big goal with a long-term perspective takes a deeper kind of confidence. This type of confidence is called *maturity*. It's a confidence that won't shatter when the day goes poorly or puff up when the day goes well, and it's also a confidence that doesn't need to put on blinders and ignore the ups and downs along the way. It transcends boys vs. girls, and it's just about what works.

you can be one thing

or two or three

you can be

the beauty *and* the beast

THE RULES

I am ashamed to admit this, but when I was a freshman in college I thought that if you went to a boy's dorm room you automatically agreed to have sex with him. As if by crossing over that little brass divider on the carpet that separates the room from the hallway, you had already committed to doing it. It was the Dorm Room Rule.

I don't know where this rule came from. I was self-aware and confident enough to know that I should never let a boy pressure or manipulate me into doing anything I didn't want to do, but at the same time, as a college freshman trying to make sense of this new environment and its social code, the Dorm Room Rule seemed like something that wasn't up to me. It felt like an unwritten rule of society, like how you need to walk quicker when someone holds the door open for you even if it's awkwardly far away. They're going to all the trouble and you don't want to seem rude or ungrateful.

As a girl, you're taught implicitly that the last thing you want is for a boy to think that you're being rude or misleading him—and this can lead down a slippery slope where you find yourself doing things you hadn't planned, all to avoid giving a bad impression to some guy you don't even know that well. I thought that if I ever broke the Dorm Room Rule, not only would I make a bad impression on the boy in question but I'd also be acting against the norms of my new college society. This is not the kind of person I should have liked to be, but it was the kind of person I was at the time—the kind of person many of us are as college freshmen trying to figure things out.

One night, after I got selected to be the newest member of the Dog Day Players, which was a very big deal—this is the same improv group that legends like Rachel Dratch and Mindy Kaling were in when they were students at Dartmouth—I wanted to celebrate. The two other freshman "puppies" and I were given MD 20/20s, otherwise known as Mad Dogs, which is technically a "flavored fortified wine." One of my fellow puppies was a guy about twice my size, so he could handle his Mad Dog, and the other was a skinny fellow who puked up his Mad Dog immediately, so he was basically sober. I've always had an iron stomach, so I kept my Mad Dog down and blacked out.

I came to and I was alone at a frat party, having somehow become separated from my group. On its own, this is not cause for panic—Dartmouth is a small community and I felt safe enough—but then, before I knew it, I was whisked upstairs by a young man who I felt fine about kissing on the dance floor but in a more sober state would not have gone upstairs with. Within moments I realized I was in his room, and I knew this was not what I had intended. But according to my rule, I had already agreed to have sex with him. He seemed to feel the same, and he blocked the door when I tried to leave.

Thankfully, I got a text from one of my best friends demanding to know where I was. She must have noticed I was missing from the dance floor and suspected what was up. I replied "up-stairs" and she told me in all caps, "LEAVE." Something clicked and I had a brief moment of clarity: LEAVE. I seized the moment and literally pushed past him to get to the door, apologizing dozens of times as I left. I felt like I was canceling a contract that had already been signed. I was grateful that I got out of there, but I felt bad about it. Rules are rules, or so I thought.

Another time, my friend Anastassia and I went on a double date with two foreign exchange students from Spain. We ate dinner and drank absinthe and the whole thing felt very mature and European. I had chemistry with one of the boys, we'll call him Elio, and I ended up going back to his room with him. We started hooking up, which led to sex, as per the Dorm Room Rule—until, in the middle of doing the thing, he told me that at that very moment I was taking his virginity. Or rather, that it had been taken five minutes ago. I was shocked and horrified that he hadn't told me beforehand. I had no idea he was a virgin—drinking absinthe didn't seem like a *virginal* thing to do. Performing this transformative act of virginity-taking attached me to Elio in a way I didn't want to be attached. My heart sank like I imagine a lobster's must when it realizes it is being boiled. It was already too late, since with virginity, it is taken instantly. I felt uncomfortable that this guy would be forever linked to me in such a monumental way. This was a total mistake, on account of me following my silly rule, and then him following his silly rule, which was to not tell someone you're a virgin until the thing is underway.

From that point forward, I tried to be more thoughtful about deciding to enter another person's room in an intimate setting. But I never revised the rule; that, I assumed, was impossible.

Rules are rules. You can't turn common practice upside down, I thought. All I could do was be extra careful about how I let things play out.

Then I met a guy named Jeremy. A dance-floor makeout at a rave turned into hanging out at the library and then semi-spontaneously meeting up again at parties. He even brought me my favorite garlic-knot pizza when I was pulling an all-nighter for a 24-hour take-home test. One night, I decided that Jeremy and I had been studying together during the day and then making out in frat basements at night often enough that I should take the next step and go to his room with him. It was my choice, and I knew what I was walking into. I was excited, actually.

But here's the thing about rules that aren't real: Not everyone follows them. When we got to Jeremy's room, he ended up stopping things before we went too far. He said that he didn't want to do *that* yet; he wanted to get to know me more first. I was shocked: This was a direct violation of the Dorm Room Rule. Jeremy and I started dating and then we got married nine years later, so you can assume the sex happened eventually. But when Jeremy broke the Dorm Room Rule I snapped awake, accepting what I had known somewhere deep down all along: It was never a real rule in the first place.

Just because I think I'm *expected* to do something doesn't mean I need to follow through. And even if I *did* follow through in the past, I am not locked into that same choice forever. Jeremy proved that to me: Guys can sometimes feel just as pressured to "perform" as girls feel pressured to "go with the flow"—and then the sex ends up happening as a mutual performance where each person is both the audience and the actor at once. But in that moment, we didn't pay attention to the rules. I realized, if there's a rule that doesn't feel right, especially if it's a rule that only lives inside my head, I can always change it.

* * *

The whole notion of questioning and changing rules is very foreign to me. I've always been a big rule person. I think my rule fixation comes from the deep place in my heart that wishes everyone would follow the rules so they won't do unpredictable shit. Rules should protect people.

After my mom died I remember wishing that there was a rule about how you aren't allowed to leave this earth just because you feel you no longer fit in. That rule would have protected my mom and it also would have protected me. It wasn't up to my mother to leave. She should have known better. I felt the number one rule of life should be that we don't get to know or choose when we die, and she broke it. She broke that rule and the consequence was that she got separated from me forever.

Maybe the whole reason I create rules for myself is to make sure I don't end up like her. Following rules is how I can be certain that I won't behave as unpredictably as she did, no matter how I feel in the moment. Rules are one of my greatest strengths: I can tell myself *You are not allowed to stop putting one foot in front of the other* and I will stick to that rule, which is one of the reasons I am the athlete that I am.

When I was very young, my dad taught me that trying hard and not giving up is the best way to achieve your goals. What else do you do when your wife leaves forever and drops you in a well of sadness with two children and no ladder? You grab the walls and climb because you know that if you don't, you might end up staying down there forever. You try hard because you must.

"Just try" was my dad's answer to everything, even when I couldn't sleep. I would get so frustrated because I wanted his actual help; I wanted him to lie in bed with me like I knew other parents did with their kids. Instead he would stand in the doorway and tell me to *just try*. He wouldn't leave, but he would never do anything more than stand there and watch me from his doorway perch. My dad knew all along that the good news and the bad news about not giving up is that it actually works. Trying was entirely up to me. And he was right: No matter what, I would always fall asleep.

When I was old enough, my dad made me go to tryouts for every sport imaginable. I wasn't always amenable to trying new things, but no matter how big a tantrum I threw, there was no turning the car around—I had to at least *try*. My father is a man of principle and it was his firm belief that kids should be kept busy, as if chasing soccer balls would also chase the grief away, or at least teach me some resilience. Through sports, my dad showed me how to approach challenge with grace, grit, and the fundamental understanding that losing is okay. In fact, losing is an ingredient of winning: Along the way to being good enough to win at something, you will inevitably lose.

When he got an idea about how something should be, it was very hard to dissuade him. I remember throwing a tantrum before basketball tryouts when I was in fourth grade but he made me go anyway and I sobbed through the entire thing. The other parents must have wondered whether my dad was pushing me too hard, but he knew this was not real pain. This was fear, and fear goes away if we just keep trying. The world can amaze us and we can amaze ourselves if we keep trying. And I knew that if I was truly miserable after giving basketball a fair chance he wouldn't force me to go back, but I *did* have to try. As it turns out, I ended up loving basketball and played all the way up until high school.

I'm incredibly impressed by how my dad wasn't fazed by anything—not by the other parents who might have been judging him for having a crybaby kid, and not by my hysterical display of tears. He was always so good at differentiating between childish tantrums and true pain. He must have known that compared to the other things we had been through, just about everything else was a sandbox. It never hurt anyone, not *really*, to get a little sand in their eyes every once in a while.

By the time I was in middle school, Always Try Hard was a major rule in my life; the core rule around which my entire identity revolved. I was the hardest worker I knew. I got so good at trying hard that everything became a game of "how hard I can try to get the thing." I think that's why I took so well to running, because success in track and cross-country is directly related to how hard you can push yourself. My softball and soccer careers also blossomed, and for years my life revolved around driving to tournaments in random towns across California with my dad, my teammates, and their parents.

I was a competitive person, but my greatest competition has always been against myself. I believed that my only limits were my own work ethic and pain tolerance. This was both a good thing and a bad thing.

The good thing was that I believed, on some level, that anything was possible. But the bad thing was that when I *wasn't* working, I felt anxious. It was as if my Always Try Hard Rule had a caveat that came with anxiety. This was not my dad's intention, to instill an anxiety-inducing rule in me, but by now it had taken on a life of its own. I think parents can try to nudge a kid in the right direction, but ultimately the parents have no control over how much momentum their initial nudge will carry and what direction the kid might take it.

Soon enough, I became a work machine fueled by anxiety. I didn't sleep well unless I knew I had tried my best that day, meaning *every* moment of my time had gone toward something productive. At Dartmouth, I meticulously planned every minute of my day to such an extent that I had to be at the next activity exactly when the previous activity ended. After college, when I was training for the 2016 Olympics and making *Tracktown*, I couldn't sleep unless I was literally too tired to keep my eyes open. Every night I would nod off in front of the editing desk with Jeremy after a full day of training. I didn't see this as a bad thing—I would feel satisfied when Jeremy turned off the computer and nudged me awake so I could brush my teeth. It felt like I was performing at my absolute maximum potential. Then I would crawl up to bed and I'd recall the pain I felt in my training run from earlier in the day and that would help me go to sleep, like a lullaby. In fact, during my workouts, I would make sure to emote out loud to a teammate (or just to myself) how much that rep hurt and how hard I had worked, all for the sake of a later Alexi who would need this evidence to fall asleep. But I knew the satisfaction was only temporary—as soon as I woke up, the anxiety would be back.

Even in the moments when I knew that I deserved to take a break from work and watch a movie, I couldn't allow myself to stop because that damn anxiety would kick in. I could never step back and see the bigger picture of what I had accomplished in a given day without feeling guilty about everything I had left to do tomorrow. And so browsing the Netflix queue would quickly turn into an email-checking session before I knew it. No matter how much I was actually accomplishing, the anxiety was always there.

After the 2016 Olympics, I was so dead set on following my Always Try Hard Rule that I forced myself to keep training without taking a break. But your body is like a pencil: If you sharpen it too much, it *will* break. You can't stay "peaked" forever; you need to recover so you can build up again for the next thing. If you recover properly, your next peak can be even higher than your last. But my rule wouldn't allow me to take any time off to recover, so I overtrained and developed a number of injuries, starting with a hamstring tendon tear that ultimately catalyzed a stress reaction in my sacrum. I had never been injured that seriously before, and to my complete horror, I physically could not train anymore. I'm not one to let a little bit of pain stop me from training, but this was like nothing I had ever experienced. I could hardly walk, let alone run.

I was desperate to find ways to work around my injury and cross-train so that I wouldn't lose fitness. But instead, one doctor after another told me that the most productive thing for me to do was rest and let my body heal itself. My initial hamstring injury had only required active rehabbing in order to heal, but my sacrum injury was different. When it comes to broken bones, time is the only cure. Being told that there was *nothing I could do* was very challenging. It was more painful than the injury itself. Being forced to do nothing felt like I was locked in jail. Anxiety and guilt overwhelmed me and I fell into a depression.

In time, with therapy, I slowly became healthy again. I saw that I needed to somehow reframe my Always Try Hard Rule and separate my work ethic from my anxiety, but I honestly wasn't sure it was possible. My anxiety felt like a heavy backpack that I wished I could put down. I understood instinctually and intellectually that it wasn't good or healthy to live this way. The problem was, I didn't know how to achieve the goals I dreamed of without letting go of my anxiety. This wasn't like the Dorm Room Rule, which seemed childish and obvious the moment I realized I knew better. That rule was easy to toss aside. My Always Try Hard Rule was something much deeper, a rule that was tied to the foundation of my post-Mom identity. If I didn't follow this rule, how could I be sure I wouldn't end up like *her*?

Then, when I read the copy of my mother's eulogy that my dad gave me as a wedding gift, I discovered the answer:

> What was Robbie running from? What made her activity so furious, such a battle between life and death? She demanded perfection for herself. Got angry at herself for not meeting exacting standards. But when it came to others, she was filled with generosity. She taught Alexi to ride a bike and tie her shoes and beginning math. She was a wonderful mother, giving, loving, devoted, but she never granted herself the pleasure of accepting that. As a mother, as in so many other roles, she demanded more of herself and saw what she was not rather than what she was.

I now understood that my mother and I both demand perfection from ourselves and we get angry when we fall short—not of any objective standard but of our own standard. And we set our standards impossibly high with a constantly moving ceiling. This is why my Always Try Hard Rule gave me so much anxiety, because it was impossible for me to ever try hard enough. I could never succeed.

This realization was a bucket of cold water to the face. I used to think that my Always Try Hard Rule was the only way to avoid becoming like my mom, but now I saw that blindly obeying this rule had in fact made me more like her than I ever wanted to be. I needed to come to a new understanding of my rule, one that could acknowledge that *trying hard* also means taking breaks and enjoying my accomplishments. Feeling anxious all the time is not a necessary ingredient to trying hard—in fact, it is limiting and dangerous.

It didn't feel good to come to this realization. Actually, it hurt. But it didn't hurt like sadness. It hurt like honesty. Honesty doesn't always feel good in the moment, but it is the kind of pain that forces you forward.

* * *

When you change or let go of a rule that you've had since childhood, it doesn't always leave so easily. My old feelings of anxiety still tried to creep in, especially when I was doing something that I would have considered unacceptable before, like watching a movie with my husband or talking on the phone with a friend. I had to remind myself that I didn't need to feel anxious anymore; that just because I'm not working in this exact moment doesn't mean that I'm not trying my best overall.

This was the hardest part, because for a long time, the Always Try Hard Rule had been a huge part of my life. It was even helpful: I highly doubt that without having it as a motivating force, my teenage self would have put in the hours at the track and in the library to get me where I am today. But now it was time to let it go. It felt like I was breaking up with a long-term boyfriend who had once been central to my existence.

My first serious boyfriend was in high school—let's call him Jack. I first noticed him in ceramics class at the beginning of my senior year. I never imagined that I'd care so much about pottery, but that ceramics class quickly became the most important part of my day. Jack was a football player who wore skater clothes. He had his ear pierced. Popular opinion was that he was hot. I figured he wasn't going to notice me on his own because I wasn't the most noticeable girl until you got to know me. Plus, we didn't roll in the same circles. He was a junior and I was a senior. He was on the football team and I was a runner and theater kid. I knew it would take some work to get his attention.

I began sitting in certain parts of the classroom where we could lock eyes while sculpting our vases, or cross paths if our paint just so happened to run out at *exactly the same time*. Each moment of successful flirtation felt satisfying, like when your baseball bat makes contact with the ball just right and you hear that cracking *plink* sound and the ball soars out to left field. I learned what kind of music Jack liked and I even began to dress a little bit like him, wearing fewer bright colors and more black. Not a day passed that I didn't think about kissing Jack. And when we were finally at the same party together, I made my move. I was a senior, dammit, and the world was about to end, which was how it felt for all of us when high school was almost over, so I was going to take everything I could from it. I moved toward him like I'd been on this earth far longer than he had. It happened in a laundry room, which is where a lot of kissing happened at high-school parties, and it was as awesome as I had imagined it would be.

Jack and I had enough chemistry to start dating, which was good because I thought we looked great together. We were madly in love and it all felt so wonderfully *high school*. What does it mean to feel *high school*? It's that feeling when everything in the world seems crazy and hard and impossible, but at the same time, anything might actually *be* possible, if that makes any sense at all. Nobody said high school had to make any sense. It's a washing machine. It is rough-and-tumble. You will come out different than you went in. You might turn pink.

Jack and I did every teenage thing that you can imagine. We learned how to drink and how to argue and how to make up and also how to have sex. When it came to a high-school-first-love-virginity-loss story, we really nailed it.

First love is a very particular kind of love. I think everlasting love, the kind you want to marry, is more like *confidence*. First love feels like *fearlessness*. First love is brave. When I fell for Jack, I was joyfully watching myself fall in love. I was falling in love with being in love.

To be in a relationship in high school is to be so *crazy in love* and scream about it in the good and the bad ways, which we did. Even our fights made us perfect for each other—this was another high-school thing, to be so opposite that it's perfect. I was optimistic and Jack was pessimistic. He thought the world was against us and I thought the world was for us. If something bad happened, he saw it as evidence that we were doomed to fail. He liked to say things like "Yeah, but see it's so fucked because . . ."

and "It *would be* cool, except . . ." We loved to wrestle with these opposing worldviews until we were so entangled we decided we could never be apart.

I was all in on Jack: We were in love, and it felt like I was exactly where I should be at that time in my life. It was very important to me to feel like I was growing up *normal* despite my challenging childhood, and this relationship was the most important indicator I had. Jack did sweet, wonderful things like ask me to prom by holding a little glass amulet over the Wishing Well at Disneyland. It had a picture of Tinkerbell and the word *Prom?* engraved on it. He made me feel like I was going to turn out okay.

At the end of our year together it was time for me to leave for college. I was moving all the way across the country to Dartmouth, and we broke up because Jack, true to form, saw a long-distance relationship as a curse we couldn't break instead of a challenge we might take on, as I saw it. I wasn't ready to give up as easily as he was.

But the thing about not giving up in a relationship is that it takes both of you to commit to facing the challenge together. Ours wasn't a bad breakup, it was a sad breakup. We sat in my Volvo outside my dad's house and said our final goodbyes before I left for college. Summer was over. I cried. And Jack gave me a mixtape with a letter that I still keep in my memory box.

When I got to Dartmouth, I was cold and alone for the first time in my life. I came from the Bay Area, where it was mild year-round, and I had not thought about how cold it could get in New Hampshire, let alone what it might feel like to be so lonely on top of being so frozen. Nobody had told me about vitamin D deficiency or seasonal affective disorder, so I was depressed for reasons I didn't understand, but then again, I was also depressed for reasons I did understand. I missed the constant text messaging, the CD mixtapes made especially for me, the sex, and most of all, the feeling of security that being with Jack gave me. With Jack I felt safe and grounded. I wasn't sure if I'd ever feel that way again.

I would spend hours stalking his social media pages and torturing myself. I'd click through Facebook photo albums again and again, stewing in my longing and jealously. I'd look back at photos of us together and feel resentment toward my old self, who surely hadn't enjoyed that moment with dear Jack as much as current me would have. Then, even worse, I'd look at newer photos. There Jack was at a party in Berkeley, and I know what goes on at these parties. There he was at homecoming with the beautiful girl who would always do Polynesian belly dances for the multicultural day at our school. Had he moved on?

But in time, I began to channel my energies elsewhere, into learning how to get good grades at this very difficult school, into running competitively again after two years away from the sport, into the improv theater group, and into making new friends. Eventually I thought about Jack less and less. I became okay, and then more than okay, and then, finally, I was great. The Alexi who was so high-school-forever attached to her boyfriend was gone; I had outgrown her. The new Alexi was thriving on her own at college. I realized that I didn't need Jack anymore to feel secure and grounded. My pain faded into nostalgia and he became a relic from my past. An Old Boyfriend.

I still bump into Jack occasionally when I go home to visit my dad—he hasn't left the Bay Area and I suspect he never will. That's okay. It doesn't make me emotional to see him like it used to those first few months after we broke up. Now I smile politely and continue on my way.

We all have Old Boyfriends in our lives—people who were once our entire world but whom we've outgrown. The same idea holds true with my rules. I thought I needed my Always Try Hard Rule to be an effective person, and maybe I did at one point, but then it was time to let that rule go. My old rule was limiting me from growing.

It's okay that Old Boyfriends mattered to us and it's okay that it hurts. It's also okay to let them go. We'll call it the Old Boyfriend Rule. It's all part of growing up.

* * *

More recently, I had an opportunity to put the Old Boyfriend Rule to the test. I was in Greece starring in a commercial for a major hotel company. I was told that this would be a long-form branded content piece about me exploring Greece and reconnecting with my ancestral country, and that it would be shot like a documentary, capturing my real experiences in an organic way. But when I got to Greece, basically everything I was told about the project turned out not to be true. The entire thing was completely staged, even more than any *fictional* film project I had ever worked on. The director would tell me exactly what to do, down to my smallest facial expressions, often standing in for me and instructing me to copy exactly what he did. I thought about complaining, but I held back because I didn't want to break one of my rules: I am always a team player, no matter what.

So instead of voicing my concerns, I tried simply to follow

directions and let go of my expectations. I had made a commitment. So what if this "documentary" was more like a puppet
show where I wasn't allowed to do *one* natural thing during our
twelve- to fourteen-hour shoot days? I am a team player, that's
the rule.

After we wrapped production in Greece, the crew came to
my house in Mammoth Lakes, California, to film some addi-
tional footage. The director said he wanted to interview me to
get some voiceover clips for the ad, but what he actually meant
was he wanted me to read a script he had written with exactly
the pacing, tone, and mannerisms he dictated. Even though I
wanted to tell him that reading off a script was not an interview,
I swallowed my words and followed my rule.

Everything about the "interview" seemed fine until we got to
the part about my mom—he had written a script that revealed
specific details about my mother's death. I had shared my personal background with his team in the early stages of the project, back when I thought this was actually going to be a
documentary, but sitting there with that script in my hand,
something felt *wrong*. I have always been protective about when
and how I share the specifics of my mom's death. Even though
the fact that she took her own life is public knowledge, it is still
up to me to decide when and how that fact comes out of my
mouth.

I told the director that I didn't feel comfortable talking about
the details of my mom's death in the context of this commercial
project, and couldn't we just say she died when I was young and
leave it at that? But he pushed back. There was an air of entitle-
ment in the way he talked to me about my own mother's suicide,
and I felt myself almost believing him—I had already given him

this story, so why not just be a team player and repeat it now for the camera?

The director and I were in my bedroom sitting on my bed. We were recording there because my bedroom is the quietest room in my house. He continued to press and I felt deeply torn. I wanted to put my foot down, but I felt an aversion to breaking my rule. It was eerily reminiscent of the Dorm Room Rule: We had already gone this far, so why not just do what was expected of me? That's when the Old Boyfriend Rule came to mind: I was allowed to outgrow and rewrite an old rule. Just because I've always been a team player in the past does not mean I need to follow that rule now, in a situation that feels wrong. I'm always allowed to *not* do things I don't want to do, whether it's something professional like giving an interview or something private like consenting to sex. I can always reevaluate as things change.

I didn't know exactly what to say to the director—how to tell him no—but then I remembered a passage from Mindy Kaling's book *Is Everyone Hanging Out Without Me?*, where she explains that if you don't want to do something, there is one way that you can definitely get out of it: Simply say that it makes you *uncomfortable*. And if Mindy could pull off a move like that, why couldn't I? The truth was, I did feel uncomfortable. Very uncomfortable. I'm very grateful that I could call on Mindy's hard-earned life lessons to save me in that moment. So I did as Mindy taught me and told the director again that I didn't feel comfortable talking about my mother that way. He was disappointed, but I held my ground. We recorded a different version of the line and the commercial turned out fine.

You're always allowed to make a new rule when you need to.

The girl in the dorm room staring at a naked boy and not wanting to go any further: Thinking she needs to stay might be a rule, but needing to leave can also be a rule. Rules that don't feel right probably are not right. My mom must have had a rule that if she couldn't be perfect, she would rather be nothing at all. I wish she could have known that we are the ones in control of our own rules. We have to know that we are the ones making choices, that *we make the rules*.

before bed decide tomorrow will be great

LOVE

There was an abundance of Disney princess films in my house when I was growing up. Maybe this was because my dad needed all the help he could get occupying the time of a little girl in the pre-iPad era, or perhaps he felt these princess films would serve as some kind of surrogate female mentorship for me, or maybe it was just because pretty much every house in America was stocked with Disney movies during the early 1990s. Regardless, I was sucked in. My blankets had Belle on them and my daydreams were about falling in love. I loved to submerge myself in the stories these Disney movies told, in dreams chased and dreams caught, both romantic and otherwise.

Beauty and the Beast made me feel like I *was* Belle, or *could be* Belle. I believed I deserved to land someone as dreamy as Belle's beast-turned-prince. Some might call this naïve, but why not believe you are as capable as a Disney princess? Why not believe in potential?

I think it was believing in potential, as the Disney princesses taught me, that enabled me to fall in love with my soulmate. Before there is love, there is potential. The potential might last only moments before it blossoms into love, as it did for my grandparents—my yiayia fell in love at first sight with my papou and married him ten days later—or it might take years. Love unfolds differently for everyone, but it always begins as potential.

If you think someone might have the potential to be the one you could love, that is the moment when you have to decide how to view that person: with skepticism or with optimism, with arms folded or with arms open. It's safer to be skeptical; you're less likely to get hurt. Optimism takes courage. You need courage to invest yourself in something that you hope can be great but might end up hurting you. It's like chasing a dream. You need to give it a chance because love, like a dream, is not something that the world hands to you. You have to be brave enough to believe in potential.

Potential can come at any time and in many forms. For me, it came in an unexpected place: in the middle of the night at an underground rave at Panarchy, an off-campus co-ed social house at Dartmouth. Panarchy's raves were notoriously wild, especially the one they'd throw during the week between final exams and graduation at the end of spring term, the so-called "senior week," when no one else was on campus besides the graduating seniors, who spent the whole time partying. I had just finished my freshman year and decided to stay and hang out.

At this rave, I started dancing with a cute boy I had seen around campus—he was a junior, so he must have been sticking around to hang out for senior week, too. We had never spoken but would always lock eyes whenever we saw each other. Dartmouth was a small enough campus where you'd generally recognize most people walking around, and if there was someone you found attractive but you didn't have mutual friends, the go-to move was to check each other out and then secretly hope for a run-in at one of the Greek houses or at some other social event, preferably with alcohol. So as the music swelled around us and sweaty couples danced with overflowing cups of beer in their hands, we gravitated toward each other and danced for all of five seconds before we started making out. This was Jeremy, the boy I'd one day marry, but at this point I didn't even know his name. Our kissing was a manifestation; it was one of those hookups that felt inevitable. This was before dating apps, which I would have loved for their ability to plan exactly how and why and when you are first seeing a potential romantic interest. But this was 2009, so we fell in love the old-fashioned way.

That night, time turned into taffy. Before I kissed Jeremy, I was under the impression that I was in control of time and that I had none to spare. But love proved me wrong. If you are someone who likes to be in total control of your time, which I respect, I suggest breaking your own rules when you find yourself confronted with potential, romantic or otherwise. Potential grows in the space you leave for it.

After we kissed that first time, my crush on Jeremy felt like it could either materialize into something more or just fizzle out. He was two years older and I was a lowly freshman. I thought maybe our makeout session had been heightened by the euphoria of the rave. Plus, by this time, every one of my girlfriends had kissed Jeremy—Jeremy liked kissing girls and people liked kissing in general at Dartmouth. Me, I also liked kissing. I've never been one to shy away from something just because everyone else likes it, too. There's a reason stuff like Top 40 music, spandex pants, and pizza are so popular. They're great. And so was Jeremy. But it was easier for me not to expect anything more than making out, like most hookups in college. Besides, I told myself, I didn't have the time for anything serious. I had a demanding work-study job so I could pay my rent, and was running varsity cross-country, performing in an improv group, and on my way to graduating at the top of my class in English. I was about to head off to an internship all the way across the country at Van Jones's green-economy nonprofit in Oakland. I didn't need any more commitments. But I still had a strong feeling about the tremendous potential right in front of me. Love is something that becomes suddenly urgent, if you let it in.

Jeremy and I went our separate ways that summer after senior week ended. But then, when we both came back to campus in the fall—his senior year, my sophomore year—we picked up right where we'd left off.

* * *

I think I fell in love with Jeremy long before I understood what it really meant. At first, we fell in love by talking about things we loved. We fell in love with *a set of mutual things*, like a Venn diagram. We met in the shared space in the middle among movies, plays, music, and poetry. What we loved most of all was seeing these things through each other's eyes.

It was easy to slip into a world together. One time, Jeremy and I spent all day in bed making up a story about two barnacles who were in love, and we were completely serious about their backstories and journeys. I was infatuated with Jeremy's commitment to the things inside our heads. If he could take a barnacle's dreams seriously, then surely he could take my dreams seriously, too. We liked to be in our own world, away from everything else, where anything was possible, creatively and otherwise. Within that world, potential was uninterrupted. I taught Jeremy how to cook. He didn't know how to sauté or make pasta. I taught him what a scallion was! We invented songs about nonsense while we cooked. If you find someone who pulls you out of the real world and makes you feel like the two of you are inside your own little snow globe, hold on to them.

It helped that Jeremy didn't know anything about track and field. We had lots in common, but not *everything* in common. I was starting to get serious about running around the time we met, and Jeremy was refreshingly unaware of what the steeplechase was or how many laps were in a 5k. Running was an uncertain dream for me, something I was exploring at my own pace. His unfamiliarity with the running world allowed me to chase my dream without it meaning anything to him beyond how happy it was making *me*. I was free to explore my potential in the running world without the pressure of anyone's expectations—just pure support.

We both loved writing. We fueled each other's ideas and found that our natural inclination was to build each other up, rather than bring each other down, which can sometimes happen in creative and romantic relationships. Anything felt possible; the answer was always *yes* or at least *maybe* before it was *no*. This is a good quality to look for and actively cultivate in any relationship, romantic or otherwise. It's just not worth it to spend your life with a "no" person. It isn't always immediately obvious when someone is a "no" person—it starts small. Instead of encouraging you when you make an effort to chase a dream, they laugh at you as if you're cute but misguided—and then before you know it, you're living a life that doesn't reflect the grandeur of your dreams, whatever they are. Even small dreams have their grandeur.

If you surround yourself with "no" people, then it is more likely that you'll become a "no" person, too. There is plenty of "no" energy in the world already, and frankly it is easier and safer to tell ourselves no before yes. This is the temptation of the "no"—it feels *safe*. Sometimes the fear of failure is a more powerful force than the desire for success because we feel, at some level, like we are protecting ourselves by not chasing our dreams. But if you're someone who wants to *do* things, you'll come to realize that chasing a dream is hard enough without also putting yourself at the disadvantage of being with a "no" person.

* * *

As if it was the most natural thing in the world, Jeremy and I dated from the fall of my sophomore year until forever. Even though we had to be long distance very early on, when I spent the winter term of my sophomore year in Los Angeles, the distance didn't stop us. Unlike my high-school boyfriend Jack, who saw long distance as an insurmountable chasm forcing us apart, Jeremy saw it as an opportunity to bring us closer together. We spoke on the phone every day I was away, sometimes for just a minute and sometimes for hours. We marveled at this thing unfolding between us. We tried to focus on being grateful that we had this chance to get to know each other as people without the distraction of all the physical stuff. Let me clarify: Hooking up is wonderful and fantastic and fun, and it absolutely brings couples closer together, but it can easily become the *only* thing that defines a relationship. I was glad that Jeremy and I had this opportunity to pause the physical aspect of our relationship for a period of time. (That said, Jeremy visited me in LA for one weekend and we stayed in the cheapest motel we could find and fit in as much sex as possible during our forty-eight hours together. Now that we live in LA, we always give the motel a fond wave whenever we drive past it.)

When we reunited after that winter term apart, it was as glorious as it was bittersweet. We knew we only had a precious few months together before Jeremy would graduate. Being long distance for one semester while you're both students is one thing, but Jeremy was now a senior in his final term—and the truth looming ahead was that if we *did* stay together until the end of the school year, we'd be facing at least two full years of long distance before I graduated, too—an unimaginable amount of time. But we resolved to not think too far ahead and to enjoy the time we had.

Dartmouth is a very sweet place to be in love. We had a wonderful spring term on campus together, full of parties and late-night study sessions and track meets and formals (like prom but with no rules), and then Jeremy graduated. This is when the *real* long-distance phase of our relationship began, and it would end up lasting for three years: two while I was finishing Dartmouth, and a third while I was doing my fifth year at the University of Oregon.

This is where our belief in potential was more important than ever. My friends were skeptical about my relationship with Jeremy—in their view, I was growing increasingly attached to a relationship that would inevitably snap under the weight of being long distance. And when all your friends feel skeptical about something, it's hard not to feel the same way. People, I've found, are wary of long-distance relationships when you're young. It is not the norm these days to take love that seriously in your late teens and early twenties. Time seems to be so precious that we are told not to waste it on something as ephemeral as a relationship.

But I knew I wasn't wasting my time. In fact, time spent *not* in a relationship with Jeremy felt like a waste, because I knew in my gut that he was the right person for me. I knew he and I probably would be together forever. I just had a feeling about it, like when you get a pair of jeans that fit so perfectly you know you will wear them until they disintegrate, and even then you will patch them and keep going. So we did the distance. I didn't mind that I missed him while we were apart. Missing someone you love can be joyful. I felt grateful in the bittersweet way.

* * *

If you're lucky, you can get more than just love out of love, although love is always enough. You know how sometimes it takes a certain person to tell you something and have it really hit home? Jeremy was the first person to recognize my creative talent and have it really mean something. I was naturally drawn to theater and writing and poetry, but I treated it like a hobby—my "real major" was going to be foreign policy with a minor in Arabic. But then Jeremy read the plays I wrote for the Dartmouth 10-Minute Play Festival and told me, in all seriousness, that he thought they were really good. He was already committed to becoming a filmmaker, the dream he'd had since he was a kid, and so coming from him, this meant something. His belief in my creative potential was invaluable.

Sometimes it can be unhealthy when you care a lot about what other people think, especially your romantic partner. But there is a difference between worrying about what your partner thinks and feeling empowered by someone you love. If the person you love is also someone you admire, then their support is powerful and nourishing. It mattered to me what Jeremy thought because he was (and still is) the person I admire most in the world. By believing in me, he made me feel like anything was possible.

During our long-distance time Jeremy and I each chased our dreams as satellite lovers, visiting each other whenever we could. We fed our potential like someone might feed a campfire. We sat around it and basked in its warm glow, talking about it, admiring it, and tending to it. We were very intentional about it all. Eventually, our friends got on board. Skepticism turned to admiration. It takes confidence to be the first two people who believe in something, whether it's love or anything else. You need to be the visionary for your own potential.

Finally, after three years of long distance, Jeremy moved to Oregon and we started our post-college life together. By this time he had finished his first indie feature film, *Tall as the Baobab Tree*, and I was just beginning my career as a professional runner. We didn't even own a spoon when we moved into our cottage studio rental, and our first night there we had to "borrow" silverware from the local café just so we could eat dinner. Slowly, we bought enough household things to fill our home with the type of miscellany you never really appreciate when you're growing up, like a rolling pin and bedside tables and a toothbrush stand. In this new world of adulthood, I liked finding things with Jeremy that could be *ours*. We thoughtfully crafted our life together like a collage.

Our game plan was to pay our bills however we could and to somehow make the most of my access to the world of elite running to make a second indie film. The film world is competitive, just as competitive as the athletic world, and so Jeremy and I combined forces and wrote a script for what would one day become *Tracktown*, an indie film set in the world of elite distance running about a girl chasing an Olympic dream. It was a movie that only we could make.

Jeremy and I had collaborated before, first on school projects like his senior thesis short film and on my one-act play *The Lonely Boy Eats Lunch with His Lunch*, and we were even co-writers on *Tall as the Baobab Tree*, but somehow this felt different. Being out in Oregon together, just the two of us untethered from our families, friends, and the Dartmouth community, made it feel like we were pioneers. We were in the *real world* now, finally chasing our dreams as adults.

We were a team in every way, juggling our creative and athletic responsibilities as a single unit. Jeremy would massage my shins before my early bedtime and then stay up late finishing script revisions. In the mornings I'd slip out for practice and then we'd reunite for a big breakfast. When we went to the Sundance Film Festival as participants in the Creative Producing Lab, a mentorship program for indie filmmakers, I specifically remember going to a party with Jeremy, and when we deemed it appropriate, I snuck out for a 5k double run in the dark in wintry Park City. I wove my way between partiers and moviegoers wearing full parkas, and when I finished my run, Jeremy met me in the bathroom and I threw my dress on over my running outfit and rejoined the party.

It sounds glamorous and romantic, and sometimes it felt that way, but in reality it mostly felt nerve-racking and uncertain. While the rest of our friends were making good money in career-path jobs, Jeremy and I were blazing our own trail down a very unpredictable terrain. It is one thing to believe in potential as a college student, but it's a whole different story to continue subscribing to this philosophy in the real world, where money and stability are at stake. The thing that most college kids don't think about when it comes to chasing a dream is the opportunity cost associated with it—we were dedicating prime years of our lives as fresh college grads toward chasing very unpredictable and competitive careers. With every month that passed, we could feel the window of opportunity for "normal" jobs closing as the postgrad time gap on our résumés grew longer and longer.

Jeremy grew up with entrepreneurial parents, so being your own boss was in his vocabulary from a young age, but my dad has worked for the same company since he graduated college. I was less prepared to wrap my mind around this new entrepreneurial life. But I didn't really have time to mull things over; we were *in it* now, hustling and scraping by from month to month, trying to focus on the path ahead rather than stress about the road not taken.

It would have been easy for us to crumble onto each other and succumb to the pressure we felt, both internally and externally, to give up on our dreams and cling to stability no matter the cost. Instead, we did whatever it took for the two of us to make one solid whole. At first our entire income came from my running, since I was being paid as a professional athlete and our creative work was not yet sustainable. But my running was never just me. Running is very much a team sport behind the scenes and Jeremy has always been there, massaging my shins before bed and making coffee in the morning. Whatever needs to get done will get done by one of us. We decided that the only way for us to succeed was to surrender all preconceived notions of individual ownership of our achievements, our workload, and our income. There is no time or space for pettiness when you are trying to get to the moon together. For us it was all-in, everything working toward a shared goal of *making it*. Potential doesn't wait for you to argue over whose name goes first on a byline—it shows its face and then scampers away like a coquettish squirrel. You've got to chase it down and grab it when you have the chance.

The question that Jeremy and I get the most often in interviews or at film screening Q&As is how we balance being professional and romantic partners. Our first response is that we are both people chasing our dreams, and of course the thing we're most excited to talk about is our latest project, and so *of course* we're going to collaborate with each other. It happens naturally. At the same time, we've had to remind ourselves that our creative projects, even though they're our passions, are still work, and that working together is not the same as spending quality time with each other. It took actually labeling these distinct types of interactions to help us find a good work-life balance.

Even for two people who spend every day together like Jeremy and I do, it is still helpful to say out loud what our intentions are for any given moment. We're either "working" or we're "connecting." We try to be intentional about when we're

doing one or the other—it's all too easy to slip into a work conversation while we're having a night out, or to start goofing off
while we're meant to be working. It's a forever work in progress. Our work-life balance has been its own journey and the
most important ingredients are communication and patience.
Having shared goals ultimately makes our relationship healthier and stronger. It feels so romantic to not know exactly what
we will be doing in a year from now, only that we'll be doing it
together.

* * *

As one year postcollege became two and then three, everything
seemed like it was on the right track: I was making a name for
myself as an athlete and against all odds Jeremy and I were close
to finishing our first co-directed movie, *Tracktown*. We were
scratching at the door to success but hadn't been let inside yet.

Before I made it to Rio in 2016, I was chasing an Olympic
dream but I was not squeezing too tight. I never expected I
would make it; it was an unlikely dream I chased with joy. On
the drive from Eugene to my final altitude-training stint in
Mammoth Lakes just a few weeks before I left for Rio, our Jeep
broke down in the middle of rural northeastern California on a
road with no cell service. After a kind farmer took us in and let
us use her family's landline, we got towed two hours away to
Susanville, the nearest town with a mechanic, and checked into
the Super 8 motel for the night. Unbeknownst to me, Jeremy
had planned to propose at a scenic waterfall during our road
trip—but our car breaking down didn't stop him. He got down
on one knee in our motel room and now I love the Super 8 for-

ever. Everything during that pre-Olympic time felt bursting with joy and possibility. Even though I didn't know how the Olympics would be, I felt excitement at the uncertainty ahead.

But after the Olympics, I became desperate for the next stage of my running career to grow and surpass the last. I was no longer a "nobody" runner, and the pressure of wanting to run faster and achieve more set me on a negative energy spiral. At the same time, Jeremy and I had just released *Tracktown* and we didn't have a new film project ready. As it turns out, post-Olympic depression for athletes and post-movie depression for directors are very similar. For the first time since college, we had no goal to sustain us. The same skepticism that my friends felt when I said I was in love with this long-distance boyfriend, that skepticism of thinking that an idea is cute but knowing it will never *really* work out, took root in our minds. Was this life sustainable? Could running and filmmaking be our actual living?

Anxiety crept in, and we both started questioning whether we were being irresponsible by deciding to follow our dreams instead of finding good, stable jobs. Our confidence in our potential was being confronted by a new adversary: fear. This was a different threat than we'd faced before. Skepticism can be brushed aside, but fear comes from inside *you*. A little bit of fear can be good sometimes, but when bad fear takes over your whole mind you stop believing in yourself. Jeremy and I started to feel more and more like our work was motivated by running away from failure instead of running toward opportunity. And being motivated by fear of failure is the surest way to fail, especially in the athletic and creative worlds. When fear is your primary motivation, you become fueled by *desperation* rather than *passion*. Desperation and passion are opposite ends of the same spectrum, but while passion is a magnetic force that attracts success and inspires people, desperation does the opposite. Jeremy and I spiraled into parallel depressive episodes. It was a perfect storm of fears and anxieties all coming to the surface at once in a massive chemical reaction.

When you're depressed, it is very hard to love yourself. When you don't love yourself, it's hard to have a healthy relationship with someone else. Sometimes in relationships, one person will be feeling down and the other person is able to lift them up. But when both people are down, it takes patience, kindness, and space. This is probably the hardest lesson we had to learn. At first, when I was in denial about my depression and Jeremy still saw depression as a choice rather than an illness, we were not being there for ourselves or for each other. It took time and therapy to learn that we couldn't support each other until we could first support ourselves.

The first step we took was to postpone our wedding while we both got the help we needed. Our wedding was scheduled for October 2017, but we pushed it to June 2018. We hoped that we'd have our lives together by then. It was a tough decision, but the relief we both felt afterward was an indication that we had done the right thing.

Jeremy and I allowed each other the space to help ourselves. We still lived together and slept together and worked together every day, but we did not try not to take on the weight of the other person's feelings, otherwise we would have collapsed. That's what our therapists were for. We checked in about our individual progress, but we respected the boundaries and responsibilities we each had for working on our own selves. Love doesn't mean you're everything to the other person all the time. It means you're honest about who you are in the moment while also staying committed to the joint potential of who you can be together.

The fact is, Jeremy and I met so young. We fell in love when I was nineteen and he was twenty-one. Our brains hadn't even finished developing yet. Each of us was bound to face this impasse at some point, that quarter-life crisis where you question everything. Ours just happened simultaneously because of the shared career we had built. Some people are single at this point, other people go through serious breakups or otherwise make drastic changes in their life, and some ignore the whole thing altogether and deal with it (or not) later in life. Jeremy and I needed to deal with our own shit, and we tried our best not to take it out on each other. We tried to acknowledge each other's emotions without judgment. We were completely vulnerable around each other, like fractions reduced to our lowest terms with absolutely nothing to hide. But even in our darkest moments, when we were being jerks to each other as we wrestled with our challenges, the underlying confidence that we'd get through this time together was always unwavering, and for that I am forever grateful. We may have lost our way but we did not lose our belief in each other or in our team. Our commitment to the *optimism of us* was our fuel.

After several months of consistent therapy and hard work, we were able to regain our emotional stability enough to pursue our goals with a renewed determination and purpose. My new partnership with Champion blossomed, and by early 2018 we were putting together our next movie, *Olympic Dreams*, which

Jeremy and I co-wrote with Nick Kroll and which Jeremy heroically directed, shot, and recorded sound on as a one-person
crew.

We got married that June, just under two years after the Rio
Olympics. At the time of our wedding, I was just barely beginning to run again without injury and we were in postproduction
on *Olympic Dreams* without any idea whether the film would be
successful or not. In short, nothing was certain in our lives—
much like before. But this time it felt different. It felt like we
had been melted down and forged into something stronger.
When we walked down the aisle, it felt like a victory lap.

a dream come true unfolds very very gradually
then all at once

FLAT CHEST
AND FREAKISHLY GNARLED FEET

I'll never forget the first time I read a film review about myself. I was in Los Angeles running on a hotel treadmill the morning after *Tracktown* had its world premiere at the LA Film Festival. I was relishing my joyful memories of the premiere and also daydreaming about the Rio Olympics, which were less than two months away. Then Jeremy walked in holding his phone with an excited look on his face: The first review of *Tracktown* had come out in *Variety*. This was a big deal—just knowing that *Variety* had written about our movie felt significant because it meant that as artists, we *existed* in a different way than we did before. Getting attention from a critic signified a milestone in my career as a performer and a writer. It meant my work had been deemed important enough to be worth someone's time.

I also felt nervous. With running, your race result is crystal clear. You finish with a place and a time that is objectively ranked alongside everybody you competed against. With movies, it's different. My result was not entirely in my own hands, nor was it as clear as the time on a race clock. I hoped people would respond to what I had made and, most important, how I had performed. I asked Jeremy to read the review to me as I continued running on the treadmill.

Jeremy began: "Pappas offsets the vanity aspect of her feature debut by sharing her personal insecurities." My heart sank, and Jeremy's smile faded as he continued. "Pappas isn't shy about revealing her flat chest and freakishly gnarled feet . . . and no self-respecting narcissist would dream of casting *SNL* star Rachel Dratch (aka 'Debbie Downer') as her on-screen mom—a choice that accentuates the Muppet-like side of Pappas' personality." The piece continued along those lines, with another highlight being when the review likened me to a "mentally disabled child."

There was no way around it: This was a *bad review*. As indie filmmakers trying earn our way into the spotlight, we were afraid. This could hurt us. My initial emotion was a sinking feeling that this critic did not believe in me. For me, there is no worse feeling than someone not believing in me.

But then, after the first wave of anxiety passed, I felt a sudden, unexpected surge of joy. I thought back to interviews with Wes Anderson where he spoke about critics misunderstanding his first film, *Bottle Rocket*. I felt like I now had something in common with him, like I was part of the "misunderstood club," too. I felt simultaneously rejected and accepted, which together made me feel sort of glamorous. I thought back to Tina Fey's and Amy Poehler's books, where they had each written about the negative press they received when they were first starting to *make it*, and I felt excited that I could relate to them now. Their examples taught me that success and criticism come hand in hand, like how you can't make bacon without the grease it leaves behind. It is not always pleasant, but it is the way of things.

I had five miles left to run on the treadmill with nothing else to think about but how delightful it was going to be now that I was making it. But as I ran, my mind kept drifting back to the part of my review that described my body. It reminded me of the way high-school boys talk with their friends about girls. It gnawed at me that the reviewer chose to focus on my physical features, describing what he felt was wrong with me in a way that no other authority figure in my life had done before. I tried to smile through this harsh realization and remind myself that *I was making it*, but I wasn't feeling good anymore. There was too much grease with my bacon.

I finished my run and reread the article, trying to figure out exactly what made me feel so weird. Then I found a comment from a reader at the bottom of the article, who said he was uncomfortable watching the sex scene because my character, Plumb Marigold, had "the body of a fourteen-year-old." My body, my real actual body, offended people. *That's* what it was. It wasn't what I said or how I performed, it was my body. I wasn't the soft feminine creature that most people were accustomed to in their leading ladies; I was "sharp and hard and angular," as the *Variety* reviewer wrote. I looked like an athlete, which I guess was offensive to him. I was skinny but I wasn't skinny like a model. I was strong but not voluptuous. According to this review, in so many words, my body didn't belong onscreen. What did the *Variety* Man want me to do? Present myself in a way that turned him on, rather than as what my character really was?

My character, Plumb, was being sexual in the way she knew how, as a female athlete existing in a state of perpetual prepubescence. While no other critics were as brazenly sexist and close-minded as the one from *Variety,* I did notice a pattern of writers using *quirky* to describe Plumb. The comedian Vanessa Bayer put it best when she said: "*Quirky* is not a compliment." In my mind, *quirky* is a catchall term that writers use when they're unsure how to classify an unusual woman. Hopefully we can develop a vocabulary to describe women in more nuanced ways.

The whole reason I made *Tracktown* was because I hadn't seen a female character on-screen that accurately captured my experience as an athlete—I was proud of Plumb. But as the *Variety* review soaked in and the *quirky*s piled up, I began to feel ashamed, both of my character and of myself. And I realized that this was getting under my skin because *I* didn't use to like my body either.

* * *

There was a time in college when my body was developing faster than my mind. Before I joined the cross-country team at Dartmouth, I hadn't run in two years and I had the body of a healthy young woman who had gone through puberty, partied with her friends, and ate whatever tasted good. But at Dartmouth, once I was training more seriously, I began transforming into an elite athlete.

My metamorphosis was slow. For my first few semesters, I never did a single long run *not* hungover. Long runs were on Sunday mornings and I was always out partying the night before. I didn't even know that a long run wasn't supposed to be that painful until my junior year when I tried staying in on Saturday night. I was amazed at how much better I felt without drinking heavily the night before. I am glad that I was able to make my way to that realization in my own time. When I stopped partying the night before practice, it was because I felt entirely ready. It was a choice, not a sacrifice.

My body grew leaner and stronger. Fat melted away and sinewy muscle took its place. My actual weight didn't change that much, but to all outward appearances it looked like I was shrinking. My boobs changed from grapefruits to crab apples. My legs transformed into tree trunks and my abs revealed themselves, stretching against my skin like meat patties in a shrink-wrapped package. I kept my period, which is a sign of health for an adult female athlete, but I looked completely different.

My eating habits also evolved, but I wasn't eating *less*—just the opposite. In fact, I was eating more than ever to meet the needs of my training. My body craved healthy foods because they fueled me longer and helped me recover better, so I gravitated toward steak, milk, and veggies instead of my previous diet of garlic-knot pizza, bagels with sausage and egg, beer, and fries. I was healthier and fitter than I had ever been.

If I stopped a few months into this transformation and maintained things from there, I would have looked like a strong, athletic girl. But being a competitive distance runner in Division 1 requires a level of fitness that goes beyond the "strong not skinny" vibe and instead pushes you into a head-turning category of strength. I wasn't a gazelle; I was a feral bobcat. I was strong *and* skinny. I fit in just fine with elite distance runners, but when I was among civilians I stood out.

I remember hooking up with guys in college and feeling embarrassed about my body, which felt more masculine than feminine. I saw myself not as a woman at all but as some kind of creature. The first time I took off my clothes in front of a boy

and revealed my new athletic body, I felt more naked than
naked. I wasn't alluring and voluptuous; I was striking and
harsh. I'd cross my arms over my muscular chest to hide it, just
like Plumb in *Tracktown*. As an athlete, I understood my body
was changing into something I should be proud of, but I also felt
dismayed because I wanted to be beautiful and feminine and
carefree—and I did *not* equate my fit body with beauty or femi-
ninity.

My new body also affected my female friendships. I came
across as intimidating and serious because my body was always
on the brink of competition, with veins and muscles showing
basically all the time. I could tell that some girls would feel self-
conscious around me, but the truth was that I felt self-conscious,
too. I stood out rather than fit in. I felt embarrassed by my hard-
edged body that was so demanding of sleep and steak.

Why was I so self-conscious about my body? Part of it was
that I was young and confused, just like any college girl—
growing, shrinking, trying, succeeding, and failing in equal
measures. I have never been as simultaneously *sure* and *unsure*
about myself as I was in college, where I would go from feeling
invincible one moment to invisible the next. On the track, I was
proud to wear just a sports bra and spandex shorts. But off the
track I'd wear baggy clothes to hide my body. I wore men's pants
and my dad's old T-shirts. I looked cute because this kind of
shapeless look was in fashion at the time, but I was wearing
these outfits for the wrong reasons. I felt sensitive about my
body because of what I suspected it said about me: that because
my wiry muscular body appeared to be uptight and intimidating, then so was I. I didn't like what I thought my body communicated about me as a person.

Sometime during college, most kids reach a turning point where they discover their niche and they "level up." They evolve from being confused and floundering to becoming the version of themselves that they'd like to be as adults. For me, that happened during my sophomore winter off-campus term in Los Angeles. I studied improv comedy at the Upright Citizens Brigade and the Second City theaters for three months and I stretched my Dartmouth grant money by living out of my car and crashing in a sleeping bag on the floor at various friends' dorm rooms at USC and UCLA. It was very different from my life back in Hanover.

Athletically, it felt like I was at a crossroads in my college career where I could either double down on my commitment to running and try to become a potentially world-class athlete, or I could phase running out of my life and focus on my other pursuits, like acting and writing. I was torn: I loved running. I especially loved being *good* at something and improving on it every season . . . but I was also tired of constantly feeling self-conscious. If I quit running, I could step back into my regular, soft, feminine body and fit in with all of my friends again. I still needed to keep up with my training while I was trying to decide what to do with myself, so I reached out to a local LA women's running club called the Janes to see if I could join them.

The Janes was a group of about ten women ranging from their twenties to late forties who ran serious weekly mileage and won all the LA races with times that would impress any athlete. But these women were also well rounded: They had jobs, families, and normal lives outside of competitive running. It was the first time I was around a group of confident adult women in an athletic situation, a far cry from my college teammates who were just as neuroses-addled as I was, in their own ways.

Every morning I'd wake up at five-thirty to meet the Janes at some faraway pier and chase the Los Angeles sun up into the sky while I listened to them talk about their lives, telling me stories that were so different from what I'd normally hear from my college teammates. I never knew women like this before— I certainly hadn't encountered women like this growing up. They looked how I imagined my older self might look. They were lean and strong, but they were also beautiful. More important, *they saw themselves as beautiful*. They emanated confidence and helped me understand that a lean, strong body was not repulsive; it was attractive. It doesn't project unlikability, as I thought before; it projects discipline. Discipline, I learned, just means making choices in favor of your goals. It doesn't mean you're un-chill; it means you know what you want.

Since all of my interactions with the Janes took place during hours outside of any normal waking time in my life, it almost felt like a dream, like stolen time. What else was I going to do between five-thirty and seven-thirty in the morning? I had nothing to lose by leaning in. I became more joyful in my pursuit of running; I'd wake up at four-thirty to make breakfast, which sometimes meant cooking enough eggs for my friend Christine (whose dorm I was staying in), who'd be coming home from her night out partying just as I was leaving for practice. I used to feel embarrassed that I was up so early to train, but now I celebrated it. This was more fun for everyone.

Just being around the Janes made me feel better about myself. These women didn't wilt with shame and self-loathing when they looked at themselves in the mirror; instead they smiled with pride at the strong bodies they had earned. I saw there existed an entire breed of healthy and athletic women who weren't any less beautiful than other women, just *different*-beautiful. The Janes was an athletic organization built by women, for women, with women at the center.

I am forever grateful to them and the gift they gave me by simply being themselves and letting me be around them. Their confidence gradually stuck to me, like I was walking through their perfume every day until it became part of my own aura. I became stunning to myself.

* * *

For all the reasons the *Variety* Man criticized *Tracktown,* I was proud of it. Plumb is someone I'd never seen represented accurately on-screen before. I'd worked hard to earn those "freakishly gnarled feet." My "flat chest" isn't actually that small compared to most distance runners, but I assume the reviewer didn't know any Olympic runners to compare me to. Most Olympic runners don't also write and star in feature films. I used to be so afraid that my athletic body would make me an outlier in Hollywood in a bad way, that I wouldn't be accepted as an actor or filmmaker because I looked like an athlete. I also worried that I would somehow be behind as an actor and filmmaker because of all the time I spent as an athlete. Shedding that imposter syndrome has taken time, and I am grateful to the mentors who helped me understand that this is simply not true.

Most impactful has been Richard Linklater, who was a very serious athlete himself—he played competitive baseball throughout high school and college, until a health condition cut his career short. I first met Rick at a film lab in Greece, and he told me that my experiences as an athlete have undoubtedly translated to my artistic career: athletes know how to fall down and get back up, how to work as a team, how to commit to a goal—all skills that are useful for acting and making movies. I am grateful that he took the time to share that wisdom and confidence with me.

Plumb might not be the typical "strong female lead" that men like the *Variety* critic were ready to embrace, but maybe one day, when enough female filmmakers grow up and create roles that portray *their* true experiences, the range of what is considered acceptable for female characters will have expanded. Maybe one day, we'll catch up with the generations-long lead that men have had to create complex, nuanced protagonists. The thing is, *this is my body*. And just because some people are shocked to see it onscreen doesn't mean it doesn't exist. It exists because *I* exist.

As a moviegoer you choose to enter an artist's habitat, not the other way around. Hopefully you feel welcomed, but it also might make you feel uncomfortable. My character in *Tracktown* made the *Variety* reviewer uncomfortable. We clearly do not come from the same world. But by crossing over from his world into mine—he did sit through the entire movie, after all—he acknowledged my existence. He experienced it. And his discomfort with my body is exactly the kind of discomfort I used to feel myself. He experienced it just by watching me. This is why Plumb Marigold exists. This is why I love to act.

In time, people started noticing *Tracktown* and celebrating what we had brought to the screen. *The Hollywood Reporter* published a glowing review and paid me the ultimate compliment by describing me as a "hard-to-resist blend of Audrey Hepburn and Joan Cusack." *New York* magazine compared the film to *Juno* and *Superbad* and called me a "cult figure for females in the era of body positivity." A few weeks later, a large distributor bought the worldwide rights and before I knew it, my flat chest and gnarled feet were on countless screens around the world, from movie theaters to airplanes. I even caught the attention of Paul Thomas Anderson, who mentioned in a 2017 interview with Bill Simmons that I gave a "fantastic performance." A few years later, when I premiered my next film, *Olympic Dreams*, at South by Southwest, I fully embraced my athletic body and wore a custom Champion dress and Gucci shoes in a style I call "athletic chic." I felt strong and glamorous and it felt like an expression of my full self. But it took a long time for me to come around to feeling good about myself in this way.

Feeling seen and understood is the most wonderful thing because it gives you the gift of confidence. I was lucky to find that with the Janes during a pivotal moment in my life. But for other people—whether they're athletes in a similar position to mine, or anyone who feels awkward in their own skin—I hope that Plumb Marigold helps them feel seen. And just maybe that extra boost of confidence will encourage them to keep chasing their dreams. That would be the most wonderful thing.

dear boy in middle school who told me i look like a "before" picture:

i'm not mad anymore. you are brilliant. i am always becoming a better me.

DAD-SAD

I feel sad for my dad sometimes and I don't know why. I think part of my dad-sadness comes from knowing that the way I behave in certain moments doesn't reflect how grateful I am for the things he gave me and gave up for me. When I was younger, my dad-sadness would flare up after I knew I was being a little shit to him, like when my mom would go the mental hospital and I'd throw a big temper tantrum to make up for all the attention-demanding I had suppressed when she was home. I couldn't help myself in the moment, but later that night or the next day I'd always feel sad. I'm sure there were plenty of days when I was a little angel to my dad, but I can't remember those as clearly. It's easier to remember ingratitudes than gratitudes.

For example, my dad has this obsession with taking pictures, though he never seems to have any intention of actually doing anything with the photographs. He's taken thousands of pictures over the years but I have yet to see a single photo album. His photography habit would make me so angry when I was growing up because we'd be in the middle of a nice conversation at dinner and he would stop and interrupt everything to take a picture instead of just enjoying the moment on its own. Like if he didn't capture it, we might forget that it ever happened, so he'd better take a picture so we can keep it forever.

I am sure it has something to do with him wanting to *keep* as many things as possible; I understand that now. He couldn't keep the person he loved most, his wife, the mother of his children, so dammit, he would keep everything else—from old newspapers he'd never read to photos he'd never look at. He collected these photos and newspapers with the best of intentions—he envisioned making a scrapbook in the time he did not have—but that didn't stop me from being a little shit about it. I'd roll my eyes and complain, if I even deigned to pose for a photo at all.

The thing is, my dad would take the picture anyway, and he always seemed very pleased. It's just like when I was really young and used to throw epic temper tantrums when I didn't want to go somewhere, like church, but we ended up going anyway and then afterward my dad would take us out to breakfast and seem so pleased with himself. I wanted my dad to *react*, but he never got mad at me. He was unaffected by my bad behavior and that made me feel even guiltier about it. Because, at my core, I felt *spoiled*. I have always felt this way because I've always understood what a tremendous burden it is to raise two kids when you're a single parent. I saw what my dad had to do to keep our lives on track.

When I first wanted to shave my legs in seventh grade, my dad and I were too awkward to really talk about it. So instead, as my brother and dad and I were pushing a shopping cart through a grocery store, my brother—who was just reaching the face-shaving age—did the brave deed of knocking two razors into our cart without even asking. My dad took note but didn't say anything. Then later that evening, with all the precision of an engineer, he taught my brother to shave his face and me to shave my legs, the three of us huddled over the same sink. My dad and I never talked about sex, but he did take me to the opening night of *Titanic* in 1998 for my eighth birthday, the midnight screening. It was just the two of us—none of my friends came because nobody's parents would let them see that movie at that age and especially not that late. The Jack and Rose scene was our sex talk. No words needed to be said—I understood, and he understood that I understood. We did things in our own time, in our own way. When I got my first period during cross-country practice in high school, my dad picked me up and we walked through the tampon section of the pharmacy with my aunt on speakerphone.

When I graduated from Dartmouth, my dad wanted to throw a party for me and invite all of our neighborhood friends. I didn't ask for a party but I understood that this was important to him. True to form, my dad waited until the night before to start preparations. I was in from out of town and trying to get sleep for a hard workout I had in the morning, but I was awoken at 2 A.M. by the sound of a whirring blender. My dad was making Greek meatballs for the party. I asked him to please stop making noise but he wouldn't—the meatballs *had* to get done! I stomped downstairs and tried to unplug the blender but he snatched it away and locked himself in the bathroom to continue blending the meatball mix. Then I screamed at my dad that I needed to sleep and it wasn't my fault he waited until the middle of the night before the party to make the damn meatballs. I was mad that he was keeping me up late, but I was also mad that he was staying up because of me. He already raised me and helped put me through college. He didn't need to stay up all night making meatballs for a graduation party. But he kept blending until the job was done, and I knew it was because he is so stubborn and so proud and loves me so much. I finally went back upstairs to bed and sure enough, I felt sad.

My heart went out to my father; I was generally mad at the unfairness of the overall situation he was in as a parent. He was my Giving Tree. I felt simultaneously frustrated and guilty about it. So I wished he would just get *mad* at me when I was being a brat. I wanted him to *yell* that I could never repay him for all he had sacrificed for me. I wanted him to admit that *he* was sad. But he never did. And the fact that he never got mad ended up making me feel sad.

I know I'm not the only one who feels sad in this way about a parent. Maybe the sadness begins the moment we are born, when we subconsciously become forever grateful to those people who made us possible. And so whenever we behave badly toward those people, even in little ways, like when I cut off a phone call with my dad too quickly, guilt rubs up against gratitude and gives birth to sadness.

I make up for my dad-sadness in a myriad of ways. I have a deep desire to make my dad feel parentally accomplished. When I think about what I'd like to give him, it's *satisfaction*—a metaphorical rocking chair that he can sit in and enjoy. The rocking chair comes in many forms. There are the big things, like bringing him in for a tour of the Olympic Village in Rio, or saying a special thank-you in front of the guests at my wedding. And there are the little things, like giving him rewards points. You know those rewards people get at the grocery store where you get discounts and free stuff when you earn enough points? My dad gets so much pleasure out of that. It makes him feel so good that I *still* use his phone number to get my groceries so that he can have the points. And these grocery points make him so fucking happy that it makes me sad.

This isn't to say that I don't still sometimes enact grown-up versions of my youthful little-shit behavior toward my dad. I have, on multiple occasions, exploded at him for not exercising or eating healthy. Unlike when I was a kid, though, we don't live in the same place anymore. We only get to spend a few days together in any given six-month period. So now my dad-sadness is compounded by self-resentment when I use even a minute of our precious time together being angry. As a rational adult, I *should* be able to tell my dad that I wish he'd exercise more and eat better without descending into an adolescent rage, but I can't help myself.

Everyone is like that—we revert back to our childhood behavior when we're around our parents. Jeremy gets this way whenever he goes home, too. I watch with amusement as he and his mom and dad slip into their old roles; even his sister gets in on it. Alliances rise and fall over bagels and lox as mini-arguments spring up over whose fault it was that we were all running late last night. This invariably ends with Jeremy getting annoyed at his parents, then saying something obnoxious, and then privately feeling sad about it later.

But there's a difference, I've found, between people with *two* parents and those with just one. We single-parented folk still have those same impulses to get annoyed at our parent, except I think we carry a heavier burden, an awareness that it's just us kids and our one parent against the world. When we storm away to our room in a fit of teenage moodiness, we don't have the comfort of knowing that on the other side of the door, our mom and dad are putting their heads together and asking, "How are we gonna deal with that kid?" Instead, we have the truth that our single parent is alone out there in the living room, maybe feeling just as lost as we are.

* * *

Whenever I meet a single dad, that person automatically seems very familiar to me. It's not that every single-dad situation is the same, of course, but there is something there that *feels* familiar, like when you smell something that reminds you of childhood but you're not exactly sure why. I have an infinite reservoir of a special kind of empathic love for single dads, particularly new ones who are just starting to wade through the shifting waters of raising children, in particular daughters, alone or partly alone. It is a big task.

Daughters to single dads can be such terrors. I admit we can be difficult. Whenever I see a dad-daughter combination out in the wild, I'll feel a little pang in my heart, in the same place where my dad-sadness resides. Even if I don't know anything about the dads or the daughters, I feel compelled to cheer them on—like when you're running down a hill and someone else passes you in the opposite direction. No matter how good an athlete they are, there is still a hill ahead for them to climb.

My single-dad empathy will flare up in the most unexpected times and places. The most memorable is when I got a phone call from Bill Hader. I had reached out to his agent to invite him to act in *Olympic Dreams*, which we'd be filming in South Korea during the 2018 Winter Olympics. I expected we'd hear from his agency, maybe, or more likely we wouldn't hear back at all.

I never expected that Bill would call me directly. I was in a heavily air-conditioned Airbnb in Scottsdale, Arizona, when my phone rang.

"Hello, is this Alexi?"

"Yes?"

"Um, this is Bill Hader?" He said it like a question.

"Hi!" I half fell out of the chair I was sitting on.

"Can you hear me okay?"

"Yes, I can!"

Bill continued, out of breath: "I'm at the top of a mountain, and it's pouring rain, and I'm wearing a Santa Claus costume. I'm on set. I'm sorry, I've never done this before. I've never . . . called someone like this. I don't normally do this. But I had to. Call you. I had to . . . I'm calling you to tell you that I can't be in your movie."

"Oh, that's okay!"

I said it like I was happy he couldn't be in my movie. Bill could have told me anything, literally anything, and it would have been okay. Just to hear his voice, to hear him say my name, was otherworldly. All I ever want is for the people I admire to believe in me and maybe give me a chance. Usually this applies to coaches and older teammates—never to famous people. It's always felt to me like celebrities live on a different planet, one I very much want to visit and maybe even live on one day, too. And when someone you have admired from afar says your *name*, the reality sets in that you are both people living here on earth and could possibly cross paths. The last time I felt like this was when I met Princess Belle at Disneyland and the world of *Beauty and the Beast* came to life and everything magic felt really *real*.

"I'm sorry, but I had to call you. I had to. I saw your movie *Tracktown* and I am obsessed. You're very talented."

My heart felt like it might explode into a thousand little fireworks. You know the kind of fireworks that burst and then burst *again*, giving birth to baby fireworks? That's how this felt. I think Bill Hader probably knows it means a lot to get a personal call from him. I felt literally nauseated with nerves and excitement knowing that he had watched an entire film I made and starred in, and that he *liked* it. I've always been a little bit self-conscious about my creative career—even though my pursuit of acting actually preceded my serious running career (I had been doing improv and theater at Dartmouth before I became competitive as a college athlete), I am aware that the world sees me as an "athlete-turned-actress." So to receive praise from someone like Bill Hader, an extremely talented actor who also didn't know anything about my athletic life before he watched *Tracktown*, meant the world to me.

Then Bill started explaining why he couldn't come to Korea with us: He had just gone through a separation from his wife and he promised his three young daughters he would take February off to be with them and he couldn't break his promise in order to be in a movie.

Bill told me: "It's sort of new to me, and I just have to be there for them, my girls."

Then I felt this thing that I couldn't help, which was to love Bill in the dad-sad way. I know he has an ex-wife who is a very involved mother to their girls, so it isn't nearly the same single-dad scenario that my father experienced. But there will still be moments when Bill and his daughters are alone, together. Moments when he will feel like a grown man in a dollhouse, or at least that's sometimes how I imagined my dad felt when he first became a single parent. I was four and my brother was eight. I had these big eyes and short hair, like a genderless nymph. Maybe my dad looked at us and felt like he was the only person on a desert island with two little aliens who never stopped crying and laughing and demanding things from him. I can't even imagine how he felt about me after my mom died—how could he ever think I'd turn out okay after that? Surely not unless he dedicated his entire life to me, which he did. It makes me feel so fucking spoiled and thankful all at once.

I sensed a quiver in Bill's voice. I recognized it as only a daughter of a single dad can: the quiver of *nervousness* or its close cousin, *fear*. Maybe Bill's daughters are angels, but no matter how angelic they are, all little girls have needs and fears. And when little girls are afraid, that's when their dads can't be. In these moments the dad needs to be the one who knows what made the noise, where the light switch is, and what comes next. I felt an impulse to tell him that everything was going to be okay and even better, it would be *great*. If what had happened for me was any indication, Bill's daughters would grow up and feel grateful for their father at every turn. They would be happy and complete. He didn't need to worry.

I don't know why I felt this kind of weird call to action, as if Bill needed me to help him believe in himself as a parent. Maybe he doesn't need anyone—or if he does, he probably has a whole stable of support around him because he's *Bill Hader* and I am completely unnecessary. But I felt compelled to say something— and it wasn't necessarily because I cared so deeply about helping Bill, but more because of the feelings this was stirring up about my own father. I really wanted to tell Bill what I could not tell my dad because I was too little and too needy at the time to help my dad in this way.

I took a deep breath before I spoke, careful not to botch this first and maybe only interaction I would ever have with him. I said, in the most gracious and subtle words I could find, that my dad had raised me on his own and that I always loved it when he took a rare day off from work to spend time with me. I think I said it because I know that at his daughters' ages, it is very possible that their ingratitudes will come out ahead of their gratitudes. Meaning, they are far more likely to complain to Bill about things they don't like than they are to express their appreciation for the things they do like. But that doesn't mean the gratitudes aren't there. And actually, those extra meals together and movie nights and lazy mornings that will come because he took time off work will mean more to his girls than he can ever know. A dad is a superhero in ways he can't possibly see in himself.

Bill said thank you, that was really cool to hear, and then he had to go back to set. After I hung up I just sat there, processing the conversation, and I was suddenly overcome by a wave of dad-sadness. I felt an urge to move back home to Alameda and organize my dad's house and teach him to exercise and help him with anything and everything he needs to live his best life. But then I realized that he wouldn't want me to do that. Because here's the thing about parents: Even if you feel like you owe them a debt of gratitude that you can never repay, *they don't want you to repay it*. You can call them more often, visit, and send handwritten notes—but you can never balance out all that they've done for you. That's not the way it works. It's not your job to assign a sadness to your parents that maybe isn't really there. Actually, the *sad* is not *sad* at all. It's just love.

Bill texted me later that day: *Thanks for the dad thing*.

It made me smile. It made me feel good that some part of my experience with my dad might matter to someone else. Just like Bill told me I had potential as an actor, I tried to do the same for him as a father. I wanted him to feel like he was on the verge of something wonderful.

dad

at times a punching bag

at times an umbrella

whether i am

monster or cinderella

you are everything

you incredible fella

YOU MAKE YOUR OWN CAPE

I ran my first marathon, the Chicago Marathon, about two years after the Rio Olympics. Those two years had been an arduous trek through depression and one injury after another. Part of me wanted to keep my first post-injury race under the radar, but another part of me wanted to craft a glorious comeback—and debuting in the marathon was a perfect way to do that. I had long thought about racing the marathon, ever since I watched my dad run a marathon when I was eight years old. We cried when he crossed the finish line because we were so proud. He was in *good pain*, and this was my first experience with good tears.

In the world of professional running, a marathon debut is a particularly momentous event, especially when it's a well-known track athlete transitioning to the marathon. The industry, press, and fans take note and all eyes are on you. My marathon debut would have been a momentous landmark in my career even if it weren't my first race in two years.

My goal was to run somewhere around 2:30, faster than the current Olympic-standard qualifying time. At my peak pre-injury fitness, hitting this time would have been definitely doable—but now I was essentially starting from scratch and I had no idea if I could get fit enough in time. The pressure was on.

I began training in July for the October race. I was starting from almost zero: I hadn't run for more than a few weeks at a time without injury since before the Olympics and now I was starting to train like an elite athlete again. The transition from not training at all to cross-training to aqua jogging and finally to running on land was as exciting as it was terrifying. I made a commitment that I would be debuting in Chicago and announced it publicly, and I really, really, *really* didn't want to reinjure myself before the big day. Those few months of training were a constant balancing act of trying to get as fit as possible before the race without getting hurt.

I made impressive progress but it wasn't possible to test myself in a way that would definitively show whether I was ready to run the time I hoped for. Typically, before an important race like this, you'll do "race simulation" workouts or even tune-up races like a local 10k, but putting in such a hard effort before the big day was too risky for me. When you're threading the needle between health and injury, an intense workout or a tune-up race can be the straw that breaks the camel's back and prevents you from getting to the start line healthy. I had to fly blind.

In the days leading up to Chicago I did all of my usual race-prep rituals: I spent time visualizing the course and imagining parts where I thought I might struggle, seeing myself push through the pain and continue. I saw myself executing the race plan I developed with my coach and excelling in this new event. Usually, visualizing helps me prepare for the aspects of a race I can predict and control, so that I can leave room for the things I can't predict or control. But no amount of visualizing could have possibly prepared me for what I was about to endure. Like losing your virginity, you can talk about the marathon all you want but it's impossible to really know what it's like until you actually do the thing.

Race morning began at five o'clock. I did a shakeout jog around a pitch-black Grant Park, where the start line was, and felt the beginnings of prerace nerves like butterflies preparing to take flight. I returned to my room, stretched, showered, and got my uniform on before heading back out to the park, now bathed in a veil of sunrise.

I toed the start line feeling like good pasta: just slightly undercooked. I was at the very front, with thousands of people behind me, all about to tackle the same monumental task together. I thought for a moment about how running is really a team sport masked as an individual sport. I love being on teams—from playing soccer in my youth to being on film sets today, I feel the greatest sense of purpose and fulfillment in team environments. And I thought about how I love running in the same way that I love acting, because even though your success in both disciplines is measured by your individual performance, you will be better and find more joy when you build others up and support those around you. Then the gun went off and the race began.

I tucked into a pack and locked into my goal pace. My nervousness had now turned into the excitement and thrill of competition, a familiar blend of jitters that were like relatives I hadn't seen in a long time: I was happy to be with them again and also a bit overwhelmed. It felt like just yesterday that I had taken my first steps running on dry land after months of cross-training, and now I was racing one of the biggest marathons in the world.

About ten miles in, I began to feel a weakness in my previously injured leg. There was a tug in my hamstring and my mobility started to decrease with each passing mile. I'd been told that it's normal to feel bad in the first half of a marathon and then warm up in the second half, but this didn't feel like a rough patch. This was different than the normal "just push through it" race pain; this was a matter of mechanical limitation where one leg would not lift as high as the other. I felt like my core engine was strong but one of my wheels wasn't turning right. Even though I was healthy in every other way, my hamstring was not ready to carry me at my goal pace for a full marathon. This limitation had never revealed itself in practice, probably because of how conservative my buildup was, and now I was forced to deal with a challenge I had not anticipated.

By now I was running several seconds per mile off-pace and I knew that hitting the Olympic standard would be impossible. The reality set in that I was not going to be able to achieve my goal. I was face-to-face with failure, and failure hurts—especially when there are sixteen miles of a marathon left to run. The marathon is a *beast*. But the middle of a race is not the time to consider your feelings. It is the time to evaluate your actions. I had a choice to make: I could either clock a time I wasn't hoping for and finish in an "embarrassing" place, or I could drop out. I thought about how ashamed I would feel to perform beneath what everyone was expecting of me. Plenty of elite runners in my position would make the choice to drop out so that they don't finish with a slow time on their record. But what would be worse, clocking a slow time or dropping out entirely?

Then I opened my ears to the voices around me. I tuned out of my own thoughts and just listened. I could hear people cheering for me, yelling, "Go Bravey!" I let those voices bolster me while I made my decision: Although I was no longer able to achieve my initial goal, I could still accomplish *a* goal. I could redefine what success would mean for me in this race. In that moment, I decided that success now meant being with the cheering crowd and my fellow runners and crossing the finish line no matter what my time and place were. I was determined not to give up. Simply continuing to put one leg in front of the other became the ultimate challenge. But despite the difficulty of it, I felt a sense of calm, like I was folding in with the thousands of people around me who all had the very same goal. I was not the only one who would be beyond proud to cross the finish line. The key was to put my ego aside and give myself permission to keep trying hard without expectation.

The kind of pain you are in when your goal is to *finish* a marathon is different than the kind of pain you are in when your goal is to *race* a marathon. When you race, you are constantly evaluating yourself compared to your surroundings and your competitors. But when all you care about is finishing, there is no competition except with yourself. The pain was not the jolting kind that I feel when I race, where I need to be prepared to accelerate to cover a move and keep myself in prime position relative to my competitors. This was more an accepting of a constant pain. Pain as a generality. Pain as a lifestyle. It is hard, but not in a way you can't handle if you focus on taking the next step, and then the next, and then the next. I tried to make each step as natural as possible and accept that it was going to take as long as it would take to get to the end.

When you're waist-deep in a tough marathon, you feel each and every second to its absolute fullest. A minute has never passed so slowly, which also means I have never appreciated what a minute is so thoroughly. I tried to savor this time rather than sit through it—just because my body was tired and aching and felt like it was only partially there didn't mean my mind couldn't be fully aware. I was producing half steps but full thoughts. I felt confidence and humility all at once.

As I pushed through one mile after the next, the best strategy I found was not to think about the end of the race at all, and to just trust that I'd know the finish line when I saw it. Chasing a dream is the same: It isn't helpful to fixate on the end result. The only thing that's in your control is the progress you're making today. You trust that, if you keep trying, you *will* come to the finish line eventually, whatever the finish line looks like for you. The end result will not always be in your hands. What *is* in your hands is the *try*.

I will never forget how I felt when I finally saw the finish line. I was in a haze, focusing only on moving forward, when suddenly it came into view. As if in a dream, lined up alongside the final straightaway were all the people I loved: my husband, my dad, my coach, my team, and even my best friend, Amanda. Fueled by their presence, I increased my effort and sped up—though perhaps only metaphorically; I don't think I could actually speed up in reality. The end-of-race sprint was impossible for me.

The moment when you cross the finish line, all of the superhuman strength and mental tricks you used to get yourself there evaporate, as if you use up your very final drops of gas in the exact moment you cross. I don't remember much from the finish line area, I only remember being given a finisher's medal and draped in one of those foil wraps that reflect sun in all directions as Jeremy and Amanda helped me walk to the recovery area. As I regained my bearings, I felt overwhelmingly proud. I knew that I still had a daunting road ahead to hit the Olympic standard time, but today didn't feel like a failure. It felt like a step. I hadn't given up today; I maintained my integrity.

The most important thing we can do with regard to our goals is to have integrity: Simply put, we should always want to try our best. I have always tried to be faithful to myself in this way. But if your ability to do your best is compromised by factors out of your control, then the meaning of "doing your best" changes: It means performing to the best of your ability within the new limitations. So even if your final result is different from what you hoped for at the start, you're still maintaining your integrity. For example, if it starts pouring rain in the middle of a race, running a slower time doesn't mean you're a failure. You can't control the weather. But if you use the rain as an excuse to try less hard, then that is a mistake. *That* is *giving up*. Trying your best doesn't mean being the best, it just means trying your best.

* * *

After the race came the media gauntlet. Immediately after recovering, all the professional athletes were shuttled to a press room where journalists could ask questions. I became nervous— even though I was proud just to have finished, the journalists would know that my time was far slower than the Olympic standard. I wasn't sure if I was allowed to be proud of myself. It is one thing to make a decision for yourself mid-race about what your goal needs to be, and another to answer to the people receiving you at the other end. I could tell that everyone was expecting me to feel upset at my result—but I reminded myself that I had *not* given up, I had simply reframed my goal. My integrity was intact. So instead of being disappointed when the reporters asked me about my time, I had a huge smile on my face.

How you talk about your experiences will dictate how you feel about them. Reframing our goals and rewriting our stories are powerful tools. Nobody can tell us how to feel about something. We can make our shortcomings into something beautiful if we want to. How we label an experience can completely change how we perceive it.

A common trait I've discovered among competitive athletes is that we never like to make ourselves feel like failures. Even if we did not meet our expectations for how a competition would go, we can see it through a lens of growth rather than failure, and in time come to feel good about ourselves. A tough race becomes a learning experience framed within the bigger picture of success. So when the interviewers in the marathon press room asked me how I felt and I said "Proud," even though there was a whole other roller coaster that led to that conclusion, *proud* was more than sufficient.

The interviewer pushed, fishing for a negative-leaning quote about my time. But I persisted in my pride and forward-thinking responses. I do not have to wear my ups and downs on my sleeve, nor do I have to give other people's expectations the time of day. I do not even have to give *my own* expectations the time of day.

I am allowed to press Pause in the moment between expectation and outcome and allow myself to decide what an experience means to me. We control and interpret our narrative in an empowering way.

Some athletes think they are being authentic or relatable by publicly wallowing in their setbacks. It is comforting, in a way, to watch people fail. But I'm not here to comfort anyone. I *always* see my failures in terms of how they can make me more successful moving forward. And that is how I want to relate to people who are interested in what I have to say, because it's true. I have failed so, *so* many times, but you might not know it because I'm always reframing my story as it unfolds, and it's always pointed toward success.

* * *

I was not always this way. It's human nature for negatives to outshine positives, and it's much easier to focus on setbacks than on successes. This is the brain's default setting, to highlight the negative. For most of my life, when I went to bed my mind would inevitably zoom in on an awkward thing I'd said or fixate on one little mistake I'd made, even if I had an otherwise great day. I think it's good to acknowledge things we want to improve on in the future, but if we allow our minds to disregard our victories and marinate in our failures, then it's easy to believe that we *are* failures. It's important to actively be mindful of the good things.

My Dartmouth coach, Olympic marathoner Mark Coogan, used to make us take a moment at the end of each run to consciously reflect on the task we'd finished before we were allowed to go into the locker room. He noticed that we'd always finish our runs right at the locker-room door and stumble into the showers as quickly as possible, not mindful of the work we had just done. So he literally drew a line on the sidewalk and told us we were not allowed to run past that point. Whether it was a long run or just a shakeout, we had to "walk it in" and enjoy what we had accomplished. I now understand the brilliance behind what Mark was making us do: By forcing ourselves to take a moment to pat ourselves on the back every day, we were teaching our brains to highlight the positive as a routine.

Today, Jeremy and I call this *relishing*. We try to take time each night before bed to relish what went well during the day, whether it was a productive meeting or a great workout or even a tasty sandwich we had at lunch. Not only does this lift our mood and cultivate more positive and success-oriented energy, it's also fun. It's fun to feel like a winner. When you feel like a winner, success is inevitable—no matter how many setbacks you experience along the way.

When I finally understood this, I began to see failure as a kind of happiness rather than something to run away from. Losses and setbacks are instructional, not damaging. Life is not about reducing our pain to nothing, it is about embracing pain and challenge as an invitation to rise and grow. The world is not objective. It's actually up to us. No single race, test, meeting, or project exists in a vacuum, because everything that happens to us is part of a larger narrative, and we can choose what that narrative is. So why not be the hero of your own story? Being a hero is a choice you can make, not a cape someone else will drape over you. You make your own cape.

i want to be brave like the first time & wise like the last time all at once

GUCCI

I like traditions. I like how traditions are things that existed before me and will outlive me and anyone who comes after me. They make me feel rooted and stable, as if I'm included in a legacy that will endure beyond the fragility of a single human life.

I've always been envious of people with big families who all live nearby so they can enact their group traditions under the watchful eyes of parents and grandparents, aunts and uncles. When I was growing up, my grandparents were far away in Atlanta, Georgia, my dad's siblings were scattered around the country, and my mom's family was all in New York, plus we didn't talk to them much anyway. My dad and brother and I were pretty much on our own in California.

Some of our traditions were gestures of classic traditions for the sake of normalcy, like how my dad would insist on cooking every single Thanksgiving dish he knew of, including the Campbell's green bean casserole where the recipe is printed on the can itself, along with my yiayia's traditional Greek meat sauce recipe, even though it was only the three of us at dinner.

But most traditions we had, we started ourselves, like playing

Wiffle ball with my best friend, Amanda, and her family every Mother's Day. Our small family thrived on tradition because it meant stability. It meant that we were *doing well*. Our traditions all revolved around sports and food, like getting hot dogs after gymnastics practice each week when I was in elementary school, or going out for Italian food in North Beach after San Francisco Giants baseball games. The baseball games themselves were also a tradition, and we were season ticket holders. Practically everyone in the left-field bleacher section was a season ticket holder, too, and we'd see them every time we went—so, in a way, bleacher section 138 was an extension of our family.

When Jeremy and I screened *Tracktown* at the San Francisco Film Festival, we went to a ramen shop on the top floor of a shopping mall in Japantown, and there was something about its sepia-toned wood paneling that felt inexplicably familiar. I called my dad and it turns out that when my brother and I were very little, our mom would bring us to Golden Gate Park every weekend and we'd always eat at that ramen restaurant after our walks. That was a tradition that sadly ended with her. But I still loved learning about it because it instantly rekindled an emotional connection to this small corner of San Francisco that had lain dormant for decades. I will always be open to surprises like this in my life. When something feels, tastes, or smells familiar, I will assume that, maybe, that's because it is.

As an adult, I'm always on the hunt for new traditions. I like to discover my favorite places wherever I go, whether it's a restaurant or a running trail or a coffee shop or even just a street, because it feels like I'm planting "tradition seeds." I'm creating dependability and stability in every new place. I've also found a way to create a shared tradition with my mother: When I moved into my own place, my dad gave me a stainless steel cooking pot that my mom had bought. Jeremy and I call it "mom's pot" and we use it to make spaghetti. I think of her every time I use it, and in this way, we have our tradition of cooking together.

One of the few other items I have that belonged to my mom is a pair of tiny Gucci shoes that I can barely squeeze my feet into. They are classic slides, somewhere between a loafer and a slipper, in caramel leather with the iconic Gucci gold clasps across the top. Because they are so old, they have slippery wood soles instead of the rubber padding like more current editions. I don't remember my mother ever actually wearing the shoes, probably because fashion was the last thing on her mind during the short period of time that I was old enough to form memories. And then they ended up hidden in my closet instead of in the donation bin with all her other belongings. The shoes remained in hiding throughout my entire adolescence, but I took them with me to college and squeezed into them on special occasions (despite my mom's feet being several sizes smaller than mine). They made me feel glamorous and comforted at the same time. My feet were cramped but my heart was full.

When I went to Italy on my honeymoon, Jeremy and I stopped by the Gucci Museum at Gucci Garden in Florence, where the brand was born. I thought it would be inspiring to soak up the sketchbooks and other early creative artifacts from such a powerful cultural institution, one that I had a connection to, however faint, through my mother.

Walking into Gucci Garden that day was like entering a world full of colorful, fanciful clothes that existed beyond my imagination. I became my little-princess self, who is always inside me but only sometimes emerges. I walked through a room filled with furs and animal-print fabrics, and another room where little projected butterflies and hummingbirds flew around the ornately painted walls, and then a room that was full of vintage Gucci suitcases stacked from floor to ceiling. There was display after display of breathtaking coats, dresses, handbags, and evening gowns, all secure in their glass cases. I felt equally delighted and intimidated, like a farm girl who somehow marries the prince and arrives at the palace feeling like this is her destiny but also that she'll never really be able to call this new place her own. As with so many feminine things I've experienced while growing up, I was on the other side of the glass—always outside peering in, imitating, adopting, projecting, but never inherently a part of it. I sensed power but I had no power.

And then I saw them: the Gucci slides. I recognized them instantly. They were my mother's shoes. They sat there modestly atop a plain white display stand. They were the original version of the classic Gucci leather slippers, the kind with old-fashioned wood soles just like my mother's, the beginning of a tradition that will never end so long as Gucci exists, which I'm sure will be forever. Suddenly I no longer felt like an outsider peering in. I owned those shoes, the same ones that were so carefully displayed here in the museum, and I owned them because I got them from my mother. I wasn't outside the glass at all; I was one in a line of women participating in a fashion tradition, a lineage that includes my mom.

That day I spent more than a month's rent, more than a plane ticket to Europe, more money than I care to admit, on new pair of Gucci shoes—in my proper size this time. I'm very happy with my purchase. At first I felt a bit silly spending so much money on something so small and material. But the shoes felt like they could be sentimental *and* practical. They'd serve me. I knew I'd wear them and they'd make me feel good every time I looked down at my feet. They'd make me feel beautiful and confident and they'd remind me of my mom in a good way. My mom didn't intend to create this tradition for me, but I was happy to finally have created a tradition that included her. Even if I had to do a bit of work to make this tradition happen, it was a tradition that we now shared. Traditions are ours to create.

As Jeremy and I left Gucci Garden, I took a Polaroid of him with the big pink shopping bag that you can only get if you shop at the museum. I will show it to our future kid when I give her or him the shoes. In that moment of giving, my child will have a luxury I never had: They'll get to experience the moment of being handed a tradition directly from their mother. They'll feel included from the start. And when I give these shoes to my child, it won't matter whether he or she likes the shoes or not. It's not about the shoes; it's about the moment of giving. It's about us being present together and exchanging something. It's like the image on the ceiling of the Sistine Chapel where God's and Adam's fingers are nearly touching. You are performing an act that connects you to something deeper, something that transcends time. We're creating a human chain.

After I snapped the Polaroid, I carefully tucked the photo into my bag for safekeeping. Then Jeremy and I walked to our favorite coffee shop, ordered our usual—cappuccino for him, Americano for me—and read our books, like we always do.

like a middle school crush

i think about my goals

more often than i like to admit

MAYA RUDOLPH

I used to have nightmares where my mom would come to me in the form of a demonic imp-like creature. It had the body of a bat and my mother's head, complete with all of her features and glowing red eyes. I called it the *devil-bat*. When I was little the devil-bat would fly into my room at least once a week and hover over my head. It would dive in close to my face but never actually touch me. This was my version of the boogeyman. But I knew to keep it secret because if my dad found out, he would think I was traumatized and then he'd feel guilty and that's the last thing I wanted, even then. And also, I knew what my dad would say: He'd explain that the bat isn't real, which I already understood but didn't like to admit because there was a part of me that liked that at least she was still *something*.

So I didn't tell anyone about her. Instead I learned how to make the bat fly away and disappear by thrashing my legs in bed as if I was running under the covers and saying "Go away" very clearly and firmly. The devil-bat would fly off every single time. It was not a gentle monster but it also wasn't anything I couldn't handle.

I don't think of the devil-bat much anymore, but I am often

reminded of it when I have to do a workout on a treadmill. Most treadmills are not designed to go Olympic-level speeds, so when I'm mid-workout I appear to be desperately thrashing and stamping like I'm trying to escape from something, and my mind goes back to kicking under the covers in an effort to chase the devil-bat away.

The night I met Maya Rudolph I was running on a hotel treadmill as fast as it could go. This hotel was in Greece, and I was there to appear in an ad for a hotel chain. I had just flown in and production was starting the next morning. It was late, but I still needed to train. The treadmill faced a large window that looked out onto a patio with Ping-Pong tables and other games. The patio was empty since it was around ten at night—but suddenly, a pack of children stepped into my view. They pressed their faces against the glass and stared at me. There were seven children in total, five girls and two boys, and they all looked to be in elementary or middle school, though one of them was much younger than the rest. I waved to them and they seemed to take this as an indication that their circus show could begin. Children are the best way to pull you out of your own head, and suddenly I was transfixed by the vaudevillian parade of kids tumbling and dancing in front of the floor-to-ceiling windows. I wondered where their parents were and why these kids were still awake so late at night.

Then, as if on cue, a man appeared and we saw each other at the exact same time. He pointed to me and waved maniacally. I recognized him but I didn't know how. To be honest, I meet a lot of men around his age in the track-and-field world, and I'm not always sure if I'm supposed to know them, or if I don't know them but they know me. He pointed to me and the kids all gathered around him and stared at me as one. I wasn't sure who was inside the fish tank looking out and who was outside looking in.

Jeremy was standing on the treadmill next to me with his laptop propped up on the cupholder like a makeshift desk, and I told him to look at this man and his entourage of kids. He looked up, his jaw dropped, and he said: "That's Paul Thomas Anderson."

The director. I returned Paul's wave and he came inside the gym along with all the children. Paul knew who I was because he had recently seen *Tracktown*, so it was a surreal moment for everyone. Nobody expects to cross paths in such an unusual place and at such an unusual time. The kids immediately encircled me, curious how an Olympic athlete exercises. I played with them while Jeremy and Paul sat together on a weights bench watching raw footage from our new movie, *Olympic Dreams*, on the laptop. And then, a few minutes later, Maya Rudolph entered the room.

Maya was calm and decompressed in a way that was surprising but not shocking, like when you realize a famous person is not a hologram but is, of course, a real breathing person. I realized that Paul and Maya are partners, and these children were mostly theirs, with a few friends mixed in. Maya and I didn't really have time to chat beyond a simple hello—the kids were buzzing through the gym, eager for my instruction. I saw that my bag of exercise bands, speed ladders, and foam balls was basically also a bag of toys. We played for hours and had the best damn night anyone's ever had in a gym.

I noticed that one of the younger children was desperately trying to keep up with the older kids but was always one step behind. When they played on an elliptical machine, pretending it was a giant rowboat, she tried to play along even though she couldn't stretch her legs far enough to reach both pedals. Younger siblings engage themselves in the self-inflicted torture of trying to be around people who are older and more in charge than they are, for which they pay dearly in the form of tears. As a younger sibling myself, I know this feeling: When I was just a bit older than this little girl, I insisted that my dad take the training wheels off my bike so I could keep up with my older brother and his friends. We were biking on the path that ran between the neighborhood and the lagoon and I lost control of my bike and barreled straight into the murky water. My brother had told me that a monster called "the Ugg" lived in the lagoon and that it would eat me if I ever fell in. So I screamed and cried and my dad jumped in to save me, even though he was wearing a suit and tie for some reason. I was beside myself because I knew my body couldn't keep up with what my mind wanted it to do. I think every younger sibling of a certain age has this feeling: They know what they want yet are tragically under-equipped to get it.

This little girl was following her brother and sisters so intently that she was doomed to crash and burn. When the meltdown happened it was not because of a fall or some other injury but because of a disagreement with two of the older girls. She wanted everyone to frog-hop instead of run their relay race. But this would never happen. She would never have the authority to dictate the actions of her older siblings and their friends. So when the older girls ran instead of frog-hopping, she burst into tears. She cried and cried and cried. It wasn't fair that the older girls weren't listening to her! And when something feels unfair to a young child, it makes her forget what she's doing, where she is, even who she is. Like most little kids, she preferred hugs to sound reasoning, and she was quickly taken into Maya's embrace.

Often, a little girl's understanding of the world revolves around her mother. I watched Maya's daughter curl into her mother's arms and it was just perfection. There is an extra energy reservoir between a mother's arms that can almost be seen, like soup steam. She fit inside Maya's lap so nicely that it seemed to me that Maya must have received mom-training on how to hug properly; I figured that she inherited her methods from her own mother, passed along like an Olympic torch. I felt the familiar pinch of melancholy I feel whenever I encounter something like this, like when you see a distant planet through a telescope: It is there but you're not there and never can be.

The concept of being a mom one day has always felt like a scary unknown for me, foreign and even dangerous. There is a shame I feel that there are things about motherhood I can't possibly know. Shame is such a powerful emotion because it stems from the feeling that something is our own fault. And the last thing I want is to have a daughter who feels the way I did growing up, a *lack* in the mother department.

The lack I felt manifested in innumerable ways. I will never forget when I was seventeen and at soccer practice, when my teammate—let's call her Phoebe—marched off the field complaining that her ovaries hurt. Concerned for her well-being, I asked Phoebe if her contact lenses were out of place and offered some eye drops from my bag. She sprang up from her keeled-over position, a mean grin on her face, and asked me where I thought ovaries were. I didn't know much about the subject or the surrounding region, lacking a female in the house to explain such things, but I was quite certain that ovaries were in the eyeballs. Phoebe almost didn't believe me, and as I sensed the gravity of my error I tried to retract my statement but it was too late: Within seconds the whole team knew about my mistake. Phoebe didn't stop there: She told her mom, who went on to spread this juicy tidbit to the rest of the team's moms hovering on the sidelines. For the entire rest of the season, one or another mom would ask me if my ovaries were feeling okay today. Sometimes it was a lone mom who approached me, giggling, but other times it was a pack of moms. They were trying to be playful, but it didn't feel that way to me. I felt like I was in the middle of this big weird joke where I didn't know the proper reaction. Did I need help? Maybe? How can someone who didn't even know where her ovaries were ever be a mom? It seemed impossible.

* * *

I woke up the next morning and thought that the previous night with Maya and her family hadn't happened. But then I looked in my bag of exercise things and they were tangled in a way that could have only been done by seven kids working together. You know how randomness is—it's hard to take steps back and recount how it happened but the result seems like perfection. I was exhausted and had a full thirteen-hour day of filming ahead of me, but I was fueled by something much more powerful than sleep. I was running on magic.

Jeremy and I met them for dinner that evening. I don't remember exactly how it came up in conversation, but I learned that Maya lost her mom when she was little, just like me. Moreover, she grew up with her dad and an older brother four grades ahead of her—*just like me*. Growing up with a dad and an older brother after your mom dies is a very specific way for a young girl to grow up. It affects the way home feels and it also affects how you relate to the world and specifically how you relate to other women. You are self-conscious but unrestricted. You are scrappy. You feel extra responsibility all the time. You overcompensate. You grow up resembling someone you don't even really know. You are aware of your own mortality. I'd never met anyone like this before. Yes, *never*. The way Maya held her daughter in her lap the previous night? That was self-taught, not inherited. Her mothering abilities came from her own instincts, not from a system of motherhood that I had been estranged from. I don't have to be afraid of what I don't yet know how to do. Regarding motherhood, maybe I will or maybe I won't, but I'll never think that I *can't*.

Discovering what Maya and I had in common was also a special moment because Maya had never met anyone like herself, either. The way we lost our moms was different, but the sense of uncertainty and overcompensation was the same. It wears off over time, but never completely, like cigarette smoke in a car.

Being with Maya felt like I was a cookie that fell into a cup of coffee and I couldn't possibly soak up enough of it. I was surrounded by the warmth of it all. I felt like she didn't feel sorry for me or overly sympathetic to me, and I appreciated that. I have always admired Maya as a performer but she looked different to me now. I am sure she looked like she always looked, but in this moment, she looked like *me*.

It takes a certain kind of confidence for me to even say this, because she is, of course, herself. But to find out we came from a similar upbringing was so encouraging—it felt like permission

to keep going because it could all turn out great. Meeting Maya
changed my understanding of what was possible. I learned that
the time to make up my mind about what is possible is never.

A few months later, back in Los Angeles, Maya and Paul invited Jeremy and me over for dinner. As it turned out, we live
one neighborhood away from each other—Maya wrote a list of
her favorite local restaurants. I keep the list on my desk. We
have gotten together a few times since, but I don't expect to become Maya's best friend. I still have lots of work to do before I
consider myself her peer. That's okay. I think of her as a sun and
I'm a small asteroid fighting to find my place in the solar system.
I'll bask in her warmth whenever I'm lucky enough to pass close
to her orbit, but for the rest of the time, it's enough to know she's
out there.

And whenever I find myself doing a workout on a treadmill,
I don't think of my mom's devil-bat anymore. I think of when I
met Maya.

eyes set on things i want ahead.

how many miles pb&j piles tears and smiles will
accrue

i'd be lying if i said i knew

but vision becomes the view.

LICE

Inspiration can come in many forms. Sometimes it is wholesome and entirely positive, like when you discover a role model or read a particularly good book—this type of inspiration gives you a gold standard to strive toward, a beacon on a hill that fills you with hope. But other times, inspiration is born of necessity, like when you are in a challenging situation that you must surmount. My most pressing challenge as a child was escaping my mother's shadow. *Not* ending up like her. But there were other challenges, too, less existential but just as urgent in the moment, that drove—and inspired—me to become who I am today.

For two years, between kindergarten and second grade, my head was infested with lice. Yes, *two years*. I had multiple generations of the things—kids, their kids, their grandkids, great-grandkids, and more. At first it started as an itch on my head, which I told my dad about on a walk to school one day. But we were running late and he was going to miss the ferry into San Francisco and so there was no time to worry about itches. Itches are small things. In our family, we always knew the difference between small things and big things. And this is why my dad is as heartbreaking as he is brilliant. The same man who so lovingly and stubbornly hand-sewed fabric name tags into every article of clothing I had because he felt that was important was also letting me go to school with an itchy scalp. I later learned that he had no idea what head lice were, being a product of growing up on an isolated company campus in Saudi Arabia—I'm sure had he been raised in America, he would have known how serious lice are. But he didn't and so he deemed my itchy scalp a problem for me to handle. He knew when to budget his own efforts as a parent and when to let me figure it out for myself.

It wasn't always pretty, and I would not advise any parent to let scalp itches go unheeded, but I understand that it was necessary for him at the time. Remember, this was only his first year as a single parent. Single parents don't get sick days and neither do their kids. I only ever remember my dad letting me miss *one* day of school in my entire childhood, during the fourth grade, and that was to go with him to opening day of the San Francisco Giants on the first day at their new stadium. Besides that, my brother and I never stayed home from school, and I think my immune system adapted to the situation because I never got sick growing up.

But this was not an ordinary childhood case of the sniffles. This was something different. I reached up and as I scratched my scalp, I felt something moving there. To my surprise, I pulled a tiny bug out from my hair. I don't remember being grossed out by it, I just remember feeling validated that I had found the source of my discomfort. I tried to show my dad, but he didn't seem to see or really register the shiny creature crawling across my finger. He was late for work and I needed to be deposited at school. It wasn't that he didn't care, he just didn't want me to miss school (a big thing) because of a bug (a small thing). He must have assumed the bug flew into my hair, or maybe he figured all the other kids at school had lice and the nurse would take care of it . . . honestly, I can't tell you what he was thinking. It was just like our Christmas tree, where having a tree in our home was a *big thing* (there were many years when we bought the tree on Christmas day), but taking it down and throwing it out was a *small thing,* and so it'd never get done. That's why we were the only house with a Christmas tree still up in April. So in my five-year-old brain, I came to the conclusion that the bugs in my hair were my responsibility. These bugs were my bugs. I didn't complain to him about my lice for a long time after that.

As the weeks went on, I would spend my days trying to learn addition and subtraction, all the while pulling little bugs out of my hair without anyone noticing. It was very satisfying to behead the lice between my fingernails and throw them on the ground. They varied in size from roughly the dimensions of a fleck of coarse black pepper to a sesame seed all the way up to, in my memory, the size of my pinky fingernail. Sometimes my friends found bugs crawling on my shoulder. I quickly flicked them off, and most of the time, nobody thought any more about it. Kids have short memories, for the most part, except for some things that they remember forever. I thought if I could hide the evidence I would be okay.

Every day when I got home from school, I would go to the bathroom, tip my head into the sink, and shake and scratch like a crazy person. When I lifted my head back up and looked into the basin, I'd typically count anywhere from ten to forty little bugs, black shapes wriggling and exposed against the stark white porcelain. I would study them with morbid fascination, then wash them down the sink and repeat the whole process. I understood that this was a gross situation to be in, but I had also come to sort of accept it as my reality—like there might be bugs in my hair forever and this would just become another part of my daily routine, like brushing my teeth. I became a *bug-having person*, very aware that other beings were living with me all the time. *At least I'm not alone,* I would think, trying to look on the bright side. But at the same time, I knew that even if this was my new normal—I prided myself on being able to adapt to anything—this was not going to be normal to my friends or teachers or anyone else, so I guarded this secret fiercely.

Then, after carrying around my little bugs for almost two months, someone discovered my secret. A girl on the playground found a bug and asked me if it was lice. I obviously lied and told her it was just a fly. But then I went home and demanded that my dad help me get rid of my infestation. Private humiliation was one thing, but being called out publicly was another matter entirely. My dad has always been sensitive to being perceived as *normal,* and by now my situation was undeniably *abnormal.* By this time, we had an au pair living with us, and he passed the lice-cleaning responsibility along to her. If hair brushing and braiding fell into the category of female things, so did this.

The number of times my hair was washed with lice shampoo and mayonnaise well exceeded the norm, and none of it worked. To this day, whenever I smell mayonnaise, I think of my bugs. The full-grown lice would die in the poisonous mayo bath that the au pair rubbed into my hair, but then there were the *eggs*, which had to be meticulously combed out with a special lice pick before they hatched and the whole cycle started over. The au pair and I tried our best, but a kindergartener and a twenty-year-old aren't necessarily the most thorough combination, and between us we never got all the eggs out. I think we were both about as vigilant with the eggs as I was with coloring between the lines: We tried, but it was just too big a task.

The lice stayed so long that they outlasted the first au pair and our new one had to take over the task. Each week I'd sit patiently as she rubbed my hair full of mayonnaise and combed the bugs out. But deep down, I knew that her efforts were futile. Because the thing is, getting each and every egg out of my wild head of hair would require a surgical level of precision and commitment. And even though the au pairs meant well, ultimately I was a little embarrassed to have them do this for me. They were not my mom and they didn't look like moms. They looked and behaved and felt more like older cousins. I was their job, not their daughter, and ultimately they did not feel like this was *their problem*. Just like when I would later go bra shopping with my dad and he would ask the ladies who worked in the store to measure me right there on the floor in front of all the other shoppers, I've always felt weird about being helped in this intimate yet swift and professional way. I felt *serviced* but not *taken care of*. My au pairs would check the box of "do the lice wash," but they wouldn't necessarily sit there for hours until every last egg was gone.

By now, the lice had survived kindergarten and nearly all of first grade. I told myself I would *not* enter second grade with lice. I was almost seven years old now, older and wiser than before. So I decided to take matters into my own hands and rid myself of lice once and for all. Carefully debugging and then de-egging myself one strand of hair at a time was something I *could* do. I figured out that the best method was to methodically pinch and drag my fingernails across each strand of hair individually so that no egg could escape unnoticed. I felt like a scientist performing an experiment on myself. And after many hours of careful sorting, pinching, and threading in my bathroom laboratory, followed by a final self-administered mayonnaise bath for good measure, I was free. And then in second grade, I got my first boyfriend, with whom I even had my first kiss. This definitely wouldn't have happened if I was too afraid to get close to anyone on account of my bugs, so I saw how my hard work paid off.

Like many things in my childhood that didn't happen in the traditional way, ridding myself of lice was ultimately my responsibility. I don't resent my dad or the au pairs for this, even though it *should not* have been my job as a first-grader to de-lice my own hair. But *shoulds* aren't useful to anyone, and as it turns out, I was perfectly capable of handling things myself.

It is easy and often comforting to assume there are *shoulds* or *supposed-tos* in the world that we can't affect or change. The au pairs were supposed to get rid of my lice. The special comb was supposed to work. The lice shampoo was supposed to kill the eggs. But it didn't. That was my reality and I could either crumble under the injustice of it or take action on my own behalf. I made the decision to get rid of *should* and take responsibility for myself. I wouldn't wish my experience with lice on anyone, but at the same time, it was thanks to my lice that I learned I could be responsible, and feeling *responsible* paves the way to feeling *capable*.

* * *

Recently, I was in a children's bookstore in Italy that doubled as a wine bar and coffee shop. I found a book on the shelf called *La Mamma* by Mariana Ruiz Johnson. I couldn't understand all the words but I understood the pictures and the gist of it. I asked the girl working at the coffee shop to translate it for me, and she told me it said: "The mother is a lot of things. She is a round thing, soft and mobile. She is a happy center, sure like the rising sun—dependable—radiant! She brought me into the world naked and little. She gave me the healthiest meals to eat . . ." And the story goes on to tell of all the wonderful things the mama gives to the baby.

Books like this press on my little-kid heart. I sometimes wonder what it would have been like if I'd had someone to help me choose my clothes for school each morning. Surely this someone would also have picked all of the lice eggs from my hair for me. Surely, with a mama like this in the house, it would have been unthinkable for me to even have lice at all. But it turns out I didn't need that person.

I can draw a direct line between the little girl cleaning lice eggs from her hair to the adult woman who crossed the finish line at the Olympics, made *Tracktown* and *Olympic Dreams*, and is writing this book. None of those things were supposed to happen. Dreams don't come true because they're supposed to; they come true because the dreamer takes it upon herself to make them happen.

For most dreams, there is no beaten path. If your dream is unconventional or unexpected or even impossible, then it's your challenge to tackle. There is only a thick forest of thorny blackberry bushes ahead, waiting for you to clear a path for yourself. It isn't easy. There will be blood, but there will also be berries.

the thing about scary things

like spiders

is that they do not scare me nearly as much

as the things i want the most.

the *want* things creep and stay

live in my mind—

a much harder place to reach and find

cannot be killed

will grow instead

unlike the spider in my bed

are not afraid

and will not flee

rather than *boo*

say *come and get me*.

FOR THOSE WHO DREAM

Whenever one of the world's best distance runners gets injured, there's a good chance that they'll be on a flight to Arizona the next day to see Dr. John Ball. This is because John is a genius. He has seen people at their very best and their very worst, moments before they win the Olympic gold and moments after a career-ending injury. Except I don't think John believes anything is career-ending, which is why he is a genius. I have gone to great lengths to see John when I need help with an injury or pain that I can't solve on my own. When I lived in Mammoth Lakes, I made the ten-hour drive multiple times, usually with Jeremy. There are two possible routes between Mammoth and Chandler, Arizona: One takes you through Joshua Tree National Park, and another goes through Las Vegas. Most often we drove through Joshua Tree, optimistically thinking I might try to run in that magical expanse, but there were other times when I was in too much pain to train at all and so Jeremy and I would drive through Las Vegas and eat at a fancy buffet instead.

When you do a therapy session with John, you learn about your body. But if you are smart and listen closely, you can also learn about your mind. John will occasionally make off-the-cuff remarks that seem casual unless you're really paying attention. One time, when he was prodding his fingers particularly deep into my calf, he said: "Very few people actually try to be great."

At first, I was taken aback. John treats some of the best athletes in the world, all of whom I imagine are always trying to be great. So how could this be true? He told me that of all the athletes he rehabilitates, only a few actually commit to the full process of permanently healing their injuries and becoming a more durable athlete. This involves specific rehab exercises, weight routines, and even lifestyle changes that need to continue long after an athlete's initial time in John's clinic. John will often see athletes for the same injury over and over because they only visit John to cross "fix injury" off their list without truly committing to the hard, unglamorous work of post-injury rehab and strengthening. They want to get better, but they're not trying hard enough. They are interested but not committed.

To be *committed* is to be dead set on achieving your goal no matter how much tedious work it takes. If you aren't committed, then you're only interested. Someone who is *interested* will dedicate some time and energy to a goal, but not enough to make it happen no matter what. It takes a certain amount of extra bravery and dedication to make the leap from interested to committed, often in the most challenging moments when nobody would blame you for quitting. The amount of hard work and the level of uncertainty it takes to be fully committed to something can be unfathomable and daunting, especially for people who have risk-averse leanings. But if you really feel your dream calling to you, then complete commitment is what it will take and nothing less.

Sometimes, people will have convinced themselves that they're committed, but in reality they're only committed just enough to check the box "tried to pursue dreams" before retreating to the safety of the backup plan. I've had so many teammates complain to me about how *hard* it is to be a professional runner, or friends vent about how *hard* it is to find their dream job, but I'm not a good shoulder to cry on. I'm someone who will take your dreams very seriously, and if you come to me with a complaint I'm going to figure out how to help you accomplish your goal. Not everyone likes it when they're confronted with the reality of what they'll need to do if they're serious about their dreams. Because the truth is, most people are really just *interested*.

There were many moments in my career when nobody would have blamed me for giving up on my Olympic dream: when I crawled on my hands and knees across the finish line in my first college championship race, tragically out of shape and finishing second to last, only beating another girl who also crawled (but I crawled faster); when I got accepted to multiple grad schools for poetry, which would have been a respectable pivot from running; and when I finished my year at the University of Oregon and realized I would not be making enough money as a runner to support myself while training for the Olympics.

When I reflect on how I've created a stable career as an athlete and filmmaker, I realize that it has come down to choosing commitment over interest at every one of those crossroads, and countless more that aren't included in this book—even though commitment is *always* the harder path to take, especially when the going gets tough. This is why so few people actually achieve the dreams they set for themselves; someone can still invest tons of time into their goals, but when they're faced with a seemingly insurmountable challenge (or an alluring alternative), they fold and take the path of least resistance. Most people innately want to avoid pain and seek out comfort, and chasing a dream means challenging the default. It breaks my heart when I see someone give up on a dream because of hardships that could have been overcome with scrappy, hard, unglamorous work. Nobody likes to hear this, but it's the truth.

* * *

The first step to *committing* is to write down your goal so that it is not just a thing floating inside of your head. This way, you're holding yourself to something tangible, and when you achieve your dream you'll have the physical proof that you were brave enough to want it in the first place. You talk about it like it's real, you take it seriously, and this makes it more inevitable. Inevitability is like momentum: It starts slowly and with difficulty, but it builds over time until it's as clear and powerful as if it always existed. Writing down your goal is the first step.

Writing down your goal is also important because it serves as a declaration of your intention for yourself and for the world. If you don't have a goal, the world might give you one. You will be like a leaf, blowing with every breeze and wholly affected by the world around you. You don't want to be a rock, either, unaffected by the world and inflexible in your thoughts. Rather, be a tree: keeping your roots firm but also being able to sense and adapt to the world around you.

If you aren't sure you're ready to commit to your goal, try this exercise that a mentor shared with me: Imagine that all of a sudden, pursuing your goal is not an option at all for you anymore. It has been magically taken away. How do you feel? If you feel relief, then you know it wasn't right for you. But if you feel heartbroken imagining a world where you can't chase your goal, then the decision to commit is clear.

Next, tell your core team about your goal. Your core team is some combination of your family, your loved ones, and your actual team and coach (if your goal is athletic). Sharing your goal in this way puts you in the brave but vulnerable position of admitting that you want something. The goal is now out in the world, breathing open air and growing into something real. Once the goal is *real,* you will undoubtedly become more accountable to it.

Then, give yourself a window of time in which you grant yourself permission to be fully dedicated to pursuing your goal. During this time, do not question the goal itself. You don't question the workout in the middle of a rep, right? You run your hardest until the rep is done and then you reassess. A great coach once told me that when the pain sets in during a workout, it takes less mental energy to push harder than it does to think about slowing down or stopping. I've found that to be true: Momentum matters, physically and mentally.

Likewise, during your predetermined window of time, work as hard as you possibly can without worrying about what comes next. If you analyze and reevaluate too much during your time window, you might unintentionally sabotage yourself. Chase your goal until the window of time is over and then check in with yourself and your core team. The exact duration of this window of time is up to you, but make sure you set a clear start and end date for it.

This leads me to the next point, and it's an important one: Don't make the window of time between check-ins too long or too short. If you try to plan too far ahead, one of two things will happen: You'll either paralyze yourself, because the end goal will seem too far away, or you'll limit yourself. If I had tried to plan, say, five years into the future after I graduated from college, I would have counted myself out of being an Olympian entirely. Instead, I only planned a year in advance, and then allowed myself the chance to outgrow my expectations and set new ones each year. The path to achieving a dream is often circuitous and hard to predict. My rule of thumb for major life dreams is to look ahead one year at a time.

Next, figure out what resources you actually need to enable yourself to fully chase your dream during your window of time. This means the tangibles and the intangibles. For my goal of making the Olympics I needed a team, a coach, a good training environment, my own living space, running gear, health insurance, and money for food. I didn't need to be rich; I just needed to have enough.

It is important to understand what you need before you step out the door toward chasing your goal because the minute you do, you'll get bombarded with every distraction in the world. There will be a million people intentionally or unintentionally telling you what they think you need to do. For me, it was hard to see my non-athlete friends making way more money early on in their "normal" careers than I was as an Olympic hopeful. But I also knew that money wasn't my goal; making an Olympic team was. When I was just turning pro, Shalane Flanagan gave me the advice that every decision I made in pursuit of my Olympic dream should revolve around one question: *Will this help me perform better?* It wasn't useful to waste time or energy worrying about making money beyond what was necessary to cover my *needs*. I needed to be safe, well-fed, and well-equipped. Only focus on what you need to take the next step.

It takes bravery to stay the course. Setbacks will happen, and likely they'll be out of your hands because you can't control the world, the future, or anybody else. But how you think about your setbacks is entirely in your control, and this is actually more important than the setback itself. For example, if you fall down on a run, instead of becoming frustrated and letting your whole practice get ruined, rewrite the narrative in your favor: You fell because you were meant to slow down and take that run easy. It's about relentlessly staying on your own team no matter what, no matter how large or small the setback.

Financial anxiety is a big reason people give up on their goals. The resources they need can feel out of reach, or the pressure of seeing everyone else around them enjoy financial stability becomes too much to bear. I sometimes admitted to my dad how hard it was to see my friends saving money after college when I was living hand-to-mouth, but he always reassured me with the story of one of his best friends at Brown, Chris Berman. Chris would go on to become one of the pioneers of ESPN and the most recognizable voice in football—but for many years after college, while my dad was working at his steady engineering job, Chris was an unknown radio announcer building his career little by little. My dad always admired Chris's passion and dedication to his dream. Chris doesn't know this, but the example he set for my father was a big help as I stayed committed to my own dream.

Chasing a dream isn't a right, it's a privilege—and it's more likely than not that, at first, it won't be financially sustainable on its own. Those who are only *interested* tend to give up when they encounter serious challenges on the financial front, while those who are *committed* find solutions. In my case, I didn't get a paid running contract right out of college, so I needed to figure out how to financially support myself while training and paying off my student loans.

For my first several months as a post-collegiate runner, I was unsponsored, meaning I was not being supported in any way to run. I worked as a volunteer assistant coach for the UO team in exchange for continued use of their facilities, and when I competed in races I wore uniforms that I designed myself with animal print or lace, and one time I even raced in a Spider-Man top. I paid for sports massages in beer, an arrangement my massage therapist (himself a retired Olympian) was kind enough to suggest, in lieu of money. I ran well and I'm proud of myself for allowing my personality to stand out during that transitional time rather than self-consciously trying to blend in. Eventually I was invited to train with the Nike Oregon Track Club Elite, but I was a "developmental athlete" without an official sponsorship contract—so while I now had coaching and a small stipend for housing and health insurance, the rest was on me. Most of the other developmental athletes stuck around for a few months with the hope that a Nike shoe contract would come—and when it didn't, they either quit training full-time or they left town to find a different training group.

But I didn't want to leave—I knew that Eugene was the absolute best place for me to pursue my Olympic dream, even though it was nerve-racking to stay there without any financial support. I reached out to a vegetable market and a butcher in town for sponsorship, where they'd give me free produce and meat in exchange for social media posts. Over time I developed similar sponsorships with a coffee roaster, a bakery, a peanut butter company, and a fish market. I also got a part-time marketing job with an athletic organization called TrackTown USA, writing articles in support of their efforts to put on events like the US Olympic Trials. I went from having nothing to having more than enough. I felt empowered to be supported by my community and more connected to the places and people around me.

One day, while I was retrieving a steak from my butcher sponsor, Long's Meat Market, a teenage girl walked in wearing a race bib. She looked like she'd been crying. I could tell that she recognized me by the way she was looking at me, so I asked her what was wrong. She told me she'd had a bad race, and even though she'd been raised as a vegetarian, now she wanted to try eating meat for the first time because she saw my many prerace steak selfies on social media.

This young woman and I kept in touch—as it turns out, she was anemic and introducing red meat into her diet was just what her body needed. She went on to win her district championships that season. I am not in the business of converting vegetarians to meat-eaters, but I was happy about the positive impact this small but meaningful connection had, forged through a local business I'd developed a relationship with out of financial necessity. I was earning my keep in Eugene, and more than just surviving, I was thriving. It felt like my dream was starting to come true bit by bit.

To be clear, the teenager who recognized me at the butcher had no idea that I literally needed my meat sponsorship in order to be able to afford steak. Did it give me anxiety to be living this way while my college friends were making steady money? Of course. Was I sure that this would all be worth it? No. I had no idea whether I'd make it to the Olympics or not. But people who are committed must suspend their disbelief. Being committed isn't about the end result; it's about giving yourself the very best chance to get there.

My developmental-athlete peers who quit running or left Eugene were baffled that I had found a way to stay and support myself while training full-time. Referring to my food sponsorships with the local businesses, they'd ask me: "How did you *get that*?"

Implicit in the way they asked their question, in the way they said *get,* was the notion that somebody handed my food sponsorships to me—as if I had found a form online somewhere that said APPLY TO LOCAL FOOD SPONSORSHIPS HERE. It was mind-blowing to them that I had blazed this trail on my own. No system existed for that—I built it myself, one cold call at a time. That is what commitment looks like. If an opportunity isn't pre-built for you, you must build it yourself.

When I shared the actual step-by-step details of how I created my food sponsorships, I noticed that it made some teammates feel awkward or even defensive. Hopefully your commitment to your goals will inspire people rather than intimidate them, but it is also true that when you try hard, it might make some people uncomfortable, and that's okay. Just remember that their feelings are not about you.

In college, I wanted to spend the summer between my junior and senior years taking improv comedy classes in New York City while also training for the fall cross-country season. It seemed impossible at first: The classes were pricey, and living in New York would not be feasible without a job or internship to cover expenses, which was a nonstarter because if I spent all my time working then I wouldn't have time to do the things I wanted to do. I looked into financial grants that Dartmouth offered for independent-study projects, but I didn't see any that remotely matched what I hoped to do. It seemed like a dead end. So I took a meeting with a faculty adviser who helped me find an answer: If I could frame my summer as a research project, then I could apply for a general research grant and that would give me all the funding I needed.

After some brainstorming and consultation with my professors, I put together a research project called Park Performance, where I'd perform my newly learned improv theater techniques in city parks and write about what it was like to be a public performer. The money I got from Dartmouth went entirely toward my food, rent, and classes, and I lived my dream in New York City. I performed regularly in Washington Square Park and I even have the permits from the Parks Department to prove it. I lived in a studio apartment in TriBeCa with three other girls and we all slept on the floor. I was only able to do it because I pushed beyond the initial impossibility and found a solution that wasn't immediately obvious.

It can feel safer to think that certain things are impossible than to believe that *just about anything is possible if you are scrappy, creative, and bold, and don't give up*—if you see barriers as things to overcome rather than reasons to quit.

Some barriers are systematic in nature, like the challenges that girls face in the distance running world when they go through puberty. Others are discriminatory based on race, sexual orientation, and a myriad of other identifiers. I recognize that I cannot speak to the difficulties of systemic barriers that I haven't faced myself. But speaking from my own experience, I believe it's best to face all barriers head-on and fight for your dreams as hard as you can, even if it seems impossible. You can either stop making excuses for yourself or you can lead a life defined by your excuses. It can be intimidating to open yourself up to this belief, and you're likely going to have to face hard questions about whether you truly want to put in the effort for something that may at first seem impossible. I say, if you want something, decisively try to get it. That beats the alternative, which is a slow-simmering regret that often reduces into bitterness. It's better to be brave than bitter.

* * *

Once you have your needs taken care of, it's time to show up and then keep showing up every single day. It's time to take your commitment seriously. It's time to do the same thing over and over. During this stage in the process you will need to plan your days, say no to ninety percent of going-out nights, say no to fifty percent of wedding invitations, say yes to naps, and make time for all the details that will add up to your dream. It's easy to feel like there's not enough time in the day, but time can be elastic. I used to leave my exercise equipment scattered around the house, on account of being too busy to pick up after myself, until one day I broke my pinky toe when I accidentally stubbed my foot on a weight I left in the living room. All of a sudden, I had time to go to the hospital and rehab my foot for the next few weeks. Finding the five minutes a day to tidy up my equipment became easy after that. "I don't have enough time" is not a useful phrase when it comes to anything related to your dream. It's okay to actively choose to do something or not, but don't blame time. Take responsibility.

It also helps to surround yourself with people who are supportive of your pursuits. Sometimes this will mean spending time with people who are not your close friends but rather are peers who are chasing similar goals as you. These are called teammates. Teammates are different from family, which you can't choose, and also different from friends, which you do choose. A teammate is a cultivated relationship revolving around shared goals. Sometimes the best teammates are not necessarily your friends. That's okay. Friends make us feel comfortable; teammates push us. When you spend the time to build a beautiful teammate relationship, it can be just as enriching as a close friendship.

Soon enough, things will get hard. It can be easy to forget how hard *hard* really is. The biggest misconception about chasing a dream is that every moment will feel fun. But that isn't how it works. When you commit to chasing your dream, think of yourself like Alice from *Alice in Wonderland:* From her perspective there were times when being in Wonderland must have been quite challenging and stressful. Alice grows and shrinks, she is sentenced to death, and she literally fills a room with her tears at one point. Alice was constantly out of her comfort zone and tackling new challenges. There was work, but there was also Wonderland.

Chasing a dream means giving a hundred percent of what you have every day. This doesn't mean every day is a success. Some days, a hundred percent of what you have doesn't amount to much. Sometimes it's a hundred percent of crap. That's okay as long as it really was a hundred percent of what you had that day. Remember the Rule of Thirds and stay consistent. Trying your best is a habit, not a skill.

During this time of trying your best, you will need to stay brave and not succumb to fear or insecurity or any of the million other things that your competitors, your friends, your family, and the world at large will throw at you. It's easy to compare yourself to other people and decide that they have it easier than you for one reason or another, and label *that* as the reason you can't succeed. But the thing is, no one chases their goal from a level playing field. It's important to stay on your own team and to understand that there are countless paths to achieving the same goal. Just because someone else appears to be in the lead early in a race doesn't mean they'll finish first. The most important thing is that *you* are thriving on your own path.

What about unexpected setbacks, like an injury or a surprise expense or a rejection? This is where a lot of people make the subtle shift from being committed to being interested, because they learn that being committed to a dream is the most work they've ever done and that the world is not fair. *The world does not owe you your dream.* If you can accept that now, you will be much better off when the reality of the effort sets in, when you are face-to-face with the millions of steps it takes to get there and the millions of opportunities to give up and allow your dream to fade into a hobby.

When you face a setback, you have to stretch your efforts and resources more than you'd like. But even when facing a setback that seems insurmountable, committed people never see it as a dead end because that is not the story they tell themselves.

We all have stories in our heads that can help us or limit us;

make sure you understand what story you're telling yourself. People who are not committed are often tempted to tell themselves the story that it was just too hard to achieve this particular goal, that they didn't get a fair chance, or any number of legitimate-seeming narratives leading to a false inevitability. Chasing your dream is hard enough; you don't need your own mind weighing you down with tempting excuses to quit. Remember, your narrative is entirely subjective and completely up to you.

Sometimes a setback shows you that you need to make a change in your approach or rethink your time frame and pivot your short-term goals. That's okay—it's all part of the learning process. Try not to beat yourself up. The only real mistake is knowing you need a change and not making it. It's only a mistake if you don't fix it. If something doesn't go your way, call it a *lesson* and adjust accordingly. This is called *recalibrating*. Once you do it, don't look back; focus on becoming the person you want to be. You are now a person who double-checks her emails before she hits Send. Or you are now a person who stretches before and after every workout. It doesn't matter that yesterday you were a person who rolled out of bed and started working out immediately, now you're someone new. You're whoever you decide you want and need to be. Sometimes that might mean just taking a moment to rest or even not making a change at all—but at least you've actively chosen to stay the course.

Last but not least, understand that a dream comes true very slowly and then all at once. Most of the time you will be in that "very slowly" period. Don't let people make you feel dumb or naïve during this time. I had plenty of friends who thought I was crazy for turning down MFA scholarships to run for the

University of Oregon, but they didn't know how that decision fit into my larger goal of being an Olympian. Most people go through their lives, or at least their careers, never truly committing to anything. It's easy for people like that to make us dream-chasers feel self-conscious, at least early on. Remember, chasing a dream goes against their basic instinct, which is to seek out safety at all costs. To them, chasing dreams is a waste of time.

But contrary to what some people might say, *chasing a dream is not a waste of time*. It's only a waste of time if you're doing it halfway. It's like going to Dr. John Ball because you're *interested* in fixing your injury, but then you're not *committed* enough to do the rehab exercises after you leave and so your injury comes back a month later. That's what gives dream-chasing a bad reputation to all the nervous parents in the world, because a lot of people who claim to be chasing their dreams are actually just interested, not committed. They take the first few steps along the path but ultimately they aren't brave enough to truly give themselves a chance at success. It's possible that you will not succeed. But then again, maybe you will.

Maybe—that word is so pregnant with possibility. *Maybe* is a blank canvas that you can paint with inevitability if you are committed. It is often unglamorous, at least from the outside. But it's brave to be committed. And I think brave is glamorous.

Pursuing a dream might seem selfish, but it's not. As long as your dream isn't hurting anyone, if you are a person chasing a dream then you are doing good in the world. You are fulfilling your destiny. You are being a Bravey and replacing *can't* with *maybe*. You are manifesting the greatest expression of yourself.

clouds wait for no one

up in the sky

but want you to reach them

and hope you will try

Epilogue

THE END OF THE BEGINNING

When my papou passed away last year, I remember watching my dad say goodbye to his father and I saw this look in my dad's eye that reminded me of me. There was sadness, but not a terrible sadness—my grandpa was more than ninety years old and had been sick for some time—it was a *yearning* sort of sadness that I immediately recognized. It was dad-sadness from a place of gratitude, like he wished he could tell his father "thank you" one more time.

After the funeral, my dad and I were in a hotel room together and I was trying to tell him in the last few moments before I needed to catch a cab to the airport that I hoped he would take better care of himself. He'd been neglecting his fitness and I wanted to tell him that he wasn't immune to the physical degeneration that my papou had faced. I expressed concern that my dad had just spent months and months managing his father's health issues, and before that he spent years raising my brother and me, and before that he spent I don't know how long trying to keep my mom alive. And now, finally, I needed to tell him to his face to please take care of himself and go to the goddamn gym three times a week.

And my dad just smiled at me with a larger than normal smile and I was perplexed—here I was chastising him and all he did was smile. It was almost farcical. I became frustrated, wondering if my dad wasn't taking me seriously or if he was just truly impenetrable. But then I realized he wasn't smiling because he was laughing at me; he was smiling because he was *proud* of me. He was so fucking proud that I was mature and stable enough to care about him in this way. It meant that I was responsible enough for myself to also feel responsible for somebody else. He was smiling because now, in this moment, he knew that I was going to be okay.

When I was of the tucking-in age and my dad used to tell me every night "You're a good kid, you know that," I think what he was really saying is that while this wasn't exactly how he planned on raising me, he was doing his best and hopefully it was all amounting to something good. As if calling me a good kid every night would make me into a good kid. I have to assume it helped, because I am here as a product of all the things, including those good-night somethings, that my dad did for me.

My dad is an engineer, and he always preferred to teach me life lessons through actions rather than words. He taught me how to throw a baseball before he taught me how to write, which is why he gave me my brother's right-handed glove before he learned I was left-handed. Sports were the best language for him to teach me how to explore "good pain," how to work hard and push myself to the limits of my body and mind without actually hurting myself, without going to the "bad pain" place.

Success as an athlete was always the best way to show my dad that I was going to be okay. Every race I competed in was my way of showing him—and myself—that we were *doing it*. We were surviving and thriving despite and maybe because of our tragic past. The Olympics were for my dad as much as they were for me.

Truthfully, running has always been a way for me to matter, which has been the most essential mandate in my life after my mom left me in the way that she did. Performing as a runner or as an actor—any kind of performance—is a way to matter. The thing about mattering in this way, though, is that it makes me feel fulfilled and lonely all at once. If the only way I can matter is by performing, then it means that my self-worth is coming from outside rather than within. If there's nobody in the audience, do I matter?

I used to think that my professional achievements might be able to satisfy the *want* that I feel, as if external accomplishments and praise would finally give me the sense of mattering that I so desperately craved. I admit that deep inside, I will always have that want. But now I understand that no matter what I do, *I matter*. I matter in this world simply because I am in this world. I am still chasing my dreams with the reckless abandon of a kid chasing an ice-cream truck, but underneath it all, I understand that I am here and that is enough.

I am okay. I am never going to end up like my mom. There were times when both my dad and I weren't sure. But now I'm sure. And I'm sure he's sure. *I am okay.* We did it. And so my dad's goofy smile in the hotel room after Papou's funeral made me cry because it is only someone who has had serious fears, probably about himself as a dad more than about me as a daughter, who could smile in *that way*. Only people who were once nervous and uncertain can feel this kind of relief, joy, and pride. We are where we are thanks to everything that happened, and where we are is good.

many things behind

many things ahead

why feel afraid

when you can be brave instead?

ACKNOWLEDGMENTS

Thank you to Jeremy. I love you. This book would not be possible without you helping me find the words.

Thank you to Dad and Kristina.

Thank you to Louis.

Thank you to my family, friends, coaches, and mentors.

Thank you to Eliza, Clio, and Whitney for believing in me.

Thank you to Maya.

Thank you to Mommy who has her copy in the sky.

Thank you to the Braveys.

BRAVEY

ALEXI PAPPAS

A Book Club Guide

QUESTIONS AND TOPICS FOR DISCUSSION

1. In Maya Rudolph's foreword, she writes about the connections between bravery and heart, humor and sadness. How did this inform your understanding of the emotional journey Alexi Pappas shares in the book? Did you see those elements in her stories, and if so, which of them resonated with you and why?

2. On the first page of the book, Pappas tells us, "All I've ever wanted in my life is to matter." How does that inform her choices throughout the book, especially as she grows up? Do you relate to that sentiment? Why or why not?

3. Throughout her life, Pappas surrounds herself with a variety of mentors, from friends and family members to coaches and role models. How do Pappas's relationships with these mentors shape her? What does she learn from them? Who would you consider your mentors? How do you view the necessity of mentorship in your own life?

4. One of the themes throughout the book is about learning and seeking support from others while also understanding how to be yourself, or, in the words of Petra, "a very big Alexi." How does Pappas address this balance in her own life? Were you able to relate to her feelings on this? Why or why not?

5. When she opens up about her post-Olympic depression, Pappas writes, "Your brain is a body part that can get injured like any other, and it can also heal like any other." Was this a new way of thinking about mental health for you? How does the theme of mental health grow and develop throughout the book, especially in terms of how Pappas sees it?

6. Pappas writes about her mother's struggles with depression, "She didn't want people to know how she felt. But now everyone's going to know. I'm going to tell them because everyone can learn from this." What lessons can be gleaned from Pappas's experience, especially with regard to her mother? Do you see any places where this shift from being guarded to practicing transparency manifests in Pappas's own life? Or in your own life?

7. On page 174, Pappas shares the Willpower Index, which she describes as a way to help budget and understand willpower. How does this index inform her sense of balance in her life? Are there parts of your own life that you recognize as falling into the draining or boosting categories?

Did this help you frame the way you approach different activities?

8. Why do you think Pappas chose to include poems and quotes throughout the book? Which of these were your favorites? How did they complement the stories in each chapter?

9. In the Epilogue, Pappas reflects on her journey from her earliest goal of wanting to matter to realizing now that "I am here and that is enough." How did you understand her development of this way of thinking? Can you point to times in your life when you have felt this way? What else do you think Pappas learned from the process of writing her own story?

10. After reading the book, what is your own personal definition of "bravey"? How has it manifested in your life?

ABOUT THE AUTHOR

ALEXI PAPPAS is an award-winning writer, filmmaker, and Olympic athlete. Her writing has appeared in *The New York Times, Runner's World, Women's Running, Sports Illustrated, The Atlantic,* and *Outside,* among other publications, and she has been profiled in *The New York Times, Sports Illustrated, New York,* and *Rolling Stone.* Pappas co-wrote, co-directed, and starred in the feature film *Tracktown* with Rachel Dratch and Andy Buckley. Most recently, she co-wrote and starred alongside Nick Kroll in *Olympic Dreams,* the first non-documentary-style movie ever to be filmed at the Olympic Games. A Greek American, Pappas holds the Greek national record in the 10,000 meters and competed for Greece in the 2016 Olympics. She lives in Los Angeles, California.

alexipappas.com
Facebook.com/thealexipappas
Twitter: @alexipappas
Instagram: @alexipappas
askbravey@gmail.com

ABOUT THE TYPE

This book was set in Granjon, a modern recutting of a typeface produced under the direction of George W. Jones (1860–1942), who based Granjon's design upon the letterforms of Claude Garamond (1480–1561). The name was given to the typeface as a tribute to the typographic designer Robert Granjon (1513–89).

RANDOM HOUSE BOOK CLUB

Because Stories Are Better Shared

Discover

Exciting new books that spark conversation every week.

Connect

With authors on tour—or in your living room. (Request an Author Chat for your book club!)

Discuss

Stories that move you with fellow book lovers on Facebook, on Goodreads, or at in-person meet-ups.

Enhance

Your reading experience with discussion prompts, digital book club kits, and more, available on our website.

Join our online book club community!

 randomhousebookclub.com

Random
House
Book Club ™

Because
Stories Are
Better Shared

RANDOM HOUSE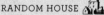